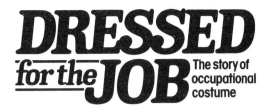

DRESSED for the JOB
The story of occupational costume

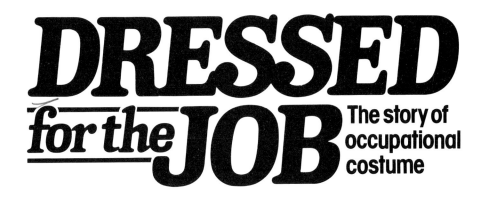

DRESSED for the JOB
The story of occupational costume

Christobel Williams-Mitchell

Illustrated by

Jeffrey J. Burn

BLANDFORD PRESS

POOLE   DORSET

First published in the U.K. 1982 by Blandford Press, Link House,
West Street, Poole, Dorset BH15 1LL.

Copyright © 1982 Blandford Books Ltd

Distributed in the United States by
Sterling Publishing Co., Inc.,
2 Park Avenue, New York, N.Y. 10016.

British Library Cataloguing in Publication Data

Mitchell, Christobel Williams
    Dressed for the job: the story of occupational
    costume.
    1. Work clothes – History
    I. Title
    391'.04   TT649

ISBN 0 7137 1020 9

Phototypeset in Linotron Garamond
by Dorchester Typesetting Group Ltd.

Printed and Bound in Great Britain by
Purnell and Sons (Book Production) Ltd., Paulton, Bristol

Contents

Acknowledgements

I WOULD LIKE TO express my gratitude first of all to Miss A. M. Buck, O.B.E. Miss Buck's kindness and scholarship are well known but can seldom have been so much appreciated as in this instance for, in spite of her many commitments, she found time to advise me and to comment on the manuscript. The help and encouragement of Dr Ann Saunders, Editor of *Costume*, have been of tremendous value too, as have her comments on the historical introduction to each chapter. Mrs Avril Lansdell's generosity in placing her own very extensive researches into occupational dress at my disposal has also been greatly appreciated.

I am also extremely grateful to the many others who have given me information and advice on both text and illustrations; in particular Miss Nancy Bradfield, Mr Frank Gerrard, M.B.E., Capt. P. E. Courage, Mr James Snowden and Miss June Swann, M.B.E.

Thanks are also due to the Automobile Association, the Institute of Meat, the Imperial War Museum, the London Transport Museum, the Museum of English Rural Life, the National Motor Museum, and the City of Westminster Cleansing Department, as well as to the staff of the Chichester Public Library, and the Library of Bishop Otter College, Chichester.

For Ewen and Jane

Introduction

THIS IS AN ACCOUNT of the clothes worn by people as they went about their ordinary, everyday occupations. These people were, for the most part, either too poor to follow fashion, or too far away from fashionable society for it to make much impression upon them.

Because this is a story that stretches from ancient times until the outbreak of the Second World War in 1939, it cannot delve very deeply into any one occupation. Furthermore, although the bulk of the material with which it deals originates in the U.K., the book also tries to show how certain basic garments appear in various countries.

Such universality is chiefly due to the fact that the great majority of people in times past were concerned, not with being fashionably dressed, but with maintaining decency and with protecting themselves from the elements as best they could. The style of many of these basic working garments, however, proved so practical that they lasted for generations—in some cases right up to the present day. Others merely served their purpose for a while and then disappeared. It is in the second category, alas, that some of the most colourful occupational costumes belong.

Another perennial type of working garment, and one that has often had very specific occupational connections, is what is known today as protective clothing—a vital part of the modern worker's life. Various kinds of apron, the most ancient of all forms of protection for the body, are as important today as they have ever been, as indeed are other garments that have existed for centuries, such as gloves and goggles.

Although those engaged in heavy manual labour that requires protective clothes may have been little influenced by changes in fashionable dress, there are, of course, certain occupations that have been— sometimes to the extent of rendering working clothes uncomfortable, inconvenient and even dangerous. Certain factories, for instance, were obliged to try to forbid the wearing of crinolines because they caught in the machinery with, occasionally, fatal results. Conversely, there have been certain occupations, particularly in the 'luxury' trades such as hairdressing, where fashionable clothes have been almost a pre-requisite. Household servants, too, who came into close contact with the wealthy and were frequently the recipients of gifts or 'castings' of fashionable garments, tended to be closer to fashion than those in most other occupations—a fact that has often been the subject of ridicule as in a poem that appeared in *Punch* in 1904 concerning the parlourmaid

Mabel. Her devotion to fashion had resulted, a short while earlier, in her having a skirt with a train that swept the ground but now, in shorter skirts—

> Her sleeves are made in open bags,
>   Like trousers in the Navy,
> No more she sweeps the street, but drags
>   Her sleeve across the gravy.

Such extravaganzas, however, were comparatively rare and for most working people styles changed slowly and were governed by utility and economy.

Although *Dressed for the Job* is mainly concerned with the clothes worn by the less affluent members of society who earned their daily bread by 'the sweat of the brow', it also refers to the use of specialized or functional dress by members of the professions. Here again, occupational costume can be divided into categories. First, the dress of lawyers and learned men, where archaic styles have been deliberately worn in order to confer dignity, makes the most of the assumption that age inspires respect—a belief which, perhaps unfortunately, has much less impact now than was once the case. The second category of professional occupational dress, of course, is the use of protective clothing for doctors and nurses, a category that really only came into being at the end of the last century.

When a book of this length covers such a broad canvas it must of necessity omit a great deal, but it is to be hoped that the reader may be stimulated to consider the subject in greater detail and, for this purpose, a list of suggested further reading has been added. To many of these books the author herself is greatly indebted. A particular mention should be made of the work of Dr Willett Cunnington, his wife Dr Phillis Cunnington and their collaborator, Miss Catherine Lucas. Their individual and joint books have provided all students of English costume not only with a vast reservoir of information but with superb examples of painstaking research and meticulous analysis.

Scholars are asked to bear with the author in her attempt to interest the general reader in a fascinating subject; and to accept at least some of its shortcomings as being due to a wish to present a general picture, in the hope that it will encourage others to delve more deeply into the story of occupational costume.

1   Tunics, not togas

Working dress in ancient times

Know you not
Being mechanical you ought not walk
Upon a labouring day without the sign
Of your profession . . .
                              Shakespeare

HOW RICH THE STREET SCENE must have looked when it was possible to glance around and see people go about their daily tasks showing 'the sign of their profession'.

As the crowds ebb and flow in the streets today one of the great tragedies of the modern world can be seen—standardization. An endless procession of a populace almost identically dressed however they earn their living. At one time people had a sense of pride in showing their occupation by the clothes they wore, now the few examples of occupational dress that remain tend to invite ridicule rather than respect. It is a sad comment on society that a person's occupation is something to be disguised rather than advertised, for when distinctive clothes are worn now it is merely to afford some special protection.

If, as the late James Laver wrote, clothes are 'the mirror of an epoch's soul' then clothes indicating occupation must surely add an extra dimension to that reflection.

To trace the story of occupational costume is to follow the way society developed, the way it created class distinctions, the way the artisan responded by a growing pride in his craft, the way the professions set themselves apart from both nobility and commonality, and the way in which changing social conditions began to erode class differences.

From ancient times clothes have been a means of emphasizing privilege and it is only comparatively recently that high fashion has become accessible to the majority. Accessible, in fact, to the working population. That is not to say that fashion does not influence working dress, it has sometimes influenced it to the point of rendering it completely impractical. But, in general, working dress has changed slowly and fashion has been the slave rather than the master of occupational costume.

The way in which working dress has lagged behind fashionable dress has partly been due to poverty, and partly to legislation in the form of what are known as sumptuary laws. These laws, though often attempts to enshrine privilege, were also used for economic reasons, such as the restriction of imports and the encouragement of exports. From medieval times there was another influence, that of the Trade Guilds, which had considerable control over what was worn by those whom today would be called 'skilled workers'.

However, overriding all these considerations, sheer practical necessity has been the main force behind the development of occupational dress—the need to have clothes that function.

Although the loincloth, the oldest garment of all, might be considered the first occupational costume, it is the tunic that has formed the basis of working dress and, in the shirt, has remained in use up to modern times.

Before the arrival of the tunic in the Mediterranean, Egyptian labourers wore the loincloth on its own, it reached only to the knee, or just above, and was probably merely twisted to keep it in place round the waist. (*Plate 1, fig. 1.*) The long loincloth worn by the upper classes never became occupational wear although, by 1500 B.C., it was fairly widely worn by household servants. Women's working garments, until the twentieth century, tended to be longer than men's, though usually shorter than current fashion. In Egypt their loincloth reached the ankle, being held in place with straps over the shoulders like wide braces. (*Plate 1, fig. 2.*) Serving girls at feasts were somewhat more briefly clad which is, of course, a tradition continued to the present day by barmaids and bunny girls. The diaphanous loincloths of the Egyptian damsels were girdled at the waist and, perhaps originating the idea of the topless waitress, their only other garment was a wide collar. Sometimes both collar and loincloth were dispensed with altogether and they were merely adorned with jewellery.

From the loincloth developed the earliest form of tunic, a length of cloth draped and tied round the body. In ancient Greece a sleeveless tunic was worn by people in all walks of life. For labourers and artisans it was a thigh-length rectangle of woollen cloth which was put round the body under one arm; front and back were pinned together on the shoulders, leaving the remaining side open. It was held together with a girdle and there was little surplus material, making it very different from the graceful folds usually associated with Greek dress. Eventually the open side was sewn, producing a cylinder which, being very narrow, was frequently fastened only on one shoulder. (*Plate 1, fig. 3.*) Two narrow rectangles, joined on top of the shoulder and down both sides, were also used to produce this tube.

Artisans often wore close-fitting caps and sometimes calf-length boots, although Homer refers to a shepherd making shoes as he required them by cutting pieces of leather and tying them round his feet. He also writes of a gardener with leather gaiters and gloves (probably resembling mittens) to protect him from brambles.

The people of Crete chose to develop the loincloth in a different way from those of Greece. Perhaps because they had learned to use leather as a medium at a very early stage in their civilisation they achieved some remarkable results. Cretan fishermen and sailors wore a loincloth, similar to that of the Egyptians with whom they traded, but labourers in the field wore a curious garment like a double apron. This fitted closely over the hips and was slightly longer at the back than the front. Unlike Egyptian workers, who went barefoot, Cretans wore leather boots and a form of gaiter. They also wore round caps like berets. During the great Minoan period (1750 B.C. to 1580 B.C.) when ladies of fashion wore the tiered skirt and open-fronted bodice, working women achieved much the same effect using a half-circle of fabric with holes on the curved edges through which they put their arms; drawing the material together with a girdle to produce an overlapping skirt.

The sleeved tunic probably came to the Mediterranean with slaves from the mountainous countries of the Middle East. T-shaped, the sleeves were originally woven as part of the garment and the shaping of the cloth to the body increased the value of the tunic as a working garment because it no longer came apart easily. As it was more convenient to work in and afforded greater protection from the elements, besides using the minimum of fabric, this tunic was widely adopted by working people.

Shepherds, always more easily recognisable by their clothes than most other working people, wore a short, rectangular cloak over the tunic and a wide-brimmed hat such as was to be worn throughout the ages by those whose work kept them out of doors in all weathers. Hair in ancient Greece was worn fairly long but slaves were easily distinguishable as they had, by law, to have theirs cut short.

Working people who did not need protection from sun and rain went bareheaded, or wore close-fitting caps. Sailors' caps were of felt or leather, with a point that fell towards the front. These may have originated in Phyrigia, part of what is now Turkey, and, in a woollen version, remained ever since a worker's garment throughout Europe. Because a cap of this type was placed on the heads of freed slaves in manumission ceremonies it was adopted as a symbol of freedom during the French Revolution.

Women workers in Greece wore a version of the fashionable tunic, the chiton; maid-servants were often as elegantly dressed as their mistresses. Male servants also seem to have taken particular care of their appearance, even to the extent of oiling their hair.

Although coloured garments of various materials were worn by wealthy Greeks, the lower classes generally retained the woollen fabric which, when not in its natural colour, was dyed with the easily available browns and greens. Costly imported dyes such as red were forbidden them.

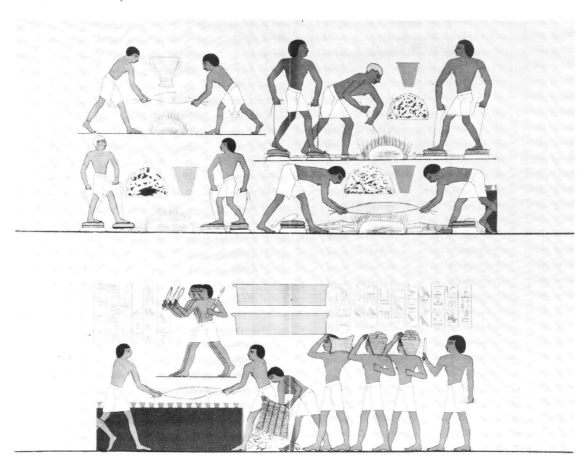

Egyptian workers in loincloths. (Eighteenth Dynasty—1580-1321 B.C.) From the tomb of Rekmire, at Thebes.

In the Roman world, as elsewhere, the earliest garment was the loincloth which, even in Imperial times, continued to be worn by slaves. The free working man wore a tunic, tied with a girdle, which came to the knee, or just above, and when strenuous work had to be done the right arm was slipped out of it completely. A similar but slightly longer tunic was worn by women who, like the men, also wore a rectangular cloak with a hood attached. More than one tunic might be worn at a time, especially during cold weather; the second tunic was eventually adopted as an under garment. (*Plate 1. fig. 4.*)

Even away from his work, the Roman labourer, should he have been able to afford it, would not have been allowed the flowing garments of the upper classes; neither were working women permitted the long robe of the Roman matron; nor were members of the 'oldest profession in the world', for Roman ladies of easy virtue had to content themselves with the shorter and less elegant *tunica*. It is possible that they may have achieved a sartorial, or should it be satirical, response by having the nails on the soles of their sandals arranged in such a way as to leave a message in the dust saying 'follow me'!

As in Greece, those exposed to the elements, like shepherds, wore wide hats, and sheepskins sometimes served them as cloaks. Among the poorer classes the use of a rectangular woollen cloak was widespread: it was sometimes dyed red and did duty also as a blanket.

One very distinctive Roman occupational costume was that of the watchmen of the Capitol—the most important temple in Rome. These men wore an adaptation of the soldiers' overtunic of leather squares, and by attaching bells to the squares they turned themselves into a perambulating alarm system.

From the fourth to the twelfth centuries, the clothes of working people changed hardly at all, although a semi-circular cloak sometimes took the place of the rectangular one. The women's undergarment remained the same, but the outer tunic was gradually replaced by a tighter short-sleeved garment, and their cloak began to be fastened in front instead of on the shoulder. For men, calf-length boots became more general, and tight-fitting trousers were sometimes worn under the tunics. These trousers were adopted from the so-called 'barbarian' dress of the northern Europeans.

As the Romans extended their Empire northwards they encountered peoples whose clothing they considered very primitive. In the first centuries after Christ the chief garment in northern Europe was the tunic. However, the trousers, of various lengths, worn underneath were a practical protection against the cold which the Roman legions were glad to adopt, although they did not make them of skins like the barbarian tribes had done from primitive times. Some peoples, including those of Ireland, wore merely a loincloth while at work with, perhaps, a rectangle of fabric over the shoulders as a cape.

Women's tunics appear to have been longer than those of men and an undertunic was worn as well, both being held together with a girdle. Along with a cloak, this was the general wear among all classes but, as Caesar writes in the account of his campaigns, working people in Gaul (roughly equivalent to modern France) were not much better than slaves, so their clothes must have been very poor indeed. For one thing there was little fabric available and for another there were few tools, even had the serf and semi-serf had the time to make himself many garments. While the great and powerful might wear the skilfully-woven 'speckled and spattered' (i.e. patterned) fabrics, there were only coarse weaves of wool and hemp for the working people.

A ninth-century monk wrote that leg bandages, strips of material wound round the leg from ankle to knee, were a distinctive mark of the Frankish workman—by this time the Franks occupied much of Europe. The bandages were apparently kept in place by the long laces of the mens' leather shoes tied about the calf.

With such a limited range of clothes, there was little to distinguish one occupation from another, though the shepherd's cloak was usually the skin of a deceased member of his flock. Like their Greek counterparts, shepherds also wore wide-brimmed hats of straw to protect them from the sun, and usually had a purse tied round their waists. Such purses, or scrips, were to remain a necessity for people who spent much of their time away from home and who had to carry food, as well as any medicines or tools they might need for the care of the sheep.

Gloves became a status symbol in later periods but they originated as a protection for those engaged in manual work and exposed to the elements; shepherds are often depicted wearing them. In Europe, in the first centuries A.D., fingerless gloves known as *mouffles* or *mitons* were used.

The withdrawal of the Roman legions from Britain and the invasions of the Northern tribes, against whom the Romans had to defend their homeland, led eventually to the downfall of Rome and to the end of the Western Empire. The Dark Ages that followed must have been especially bleak for the labouring people, particularly in North-west Europe. The Eastern Empire, which separated from the West in A.D. 285, remained a centre of culture and eventually began to exert a modifying effect on the barbarian tribes and on their clothes.

Two rulers in the Dark Ages who had a considerable influence on the lives of working people were Charlemagne, the king of the Franks, who by the time he was crowned Emperor in Rome in A.D. 800 already ruled over much of Western Europe, and Alfred the Great, the first king of England.

Charlemagne set about organizing trade, and encouraged craft and learning, at the same time as subduing many of the barbaric tribes. Alfred, who had succeeded in unifying a large part of Britain and in defeating the Danish invaders, also made great efforts to encourage culture. Craftsmen flocked to both their courts, bettering the status of artisans as well as their skills. One result was that tools improved which in turn improved the workmanship of clothes.

Towns were developing and such cities as already existed were getting larger, though life in them was rural and was to remain so for centuries. Many craftsmen lived in these towns and cities, early manuscripts show them at work wearing simple belted tunics with drawers underneath; these were merely rectangles of cloth passed between the legs and held in place round the waist by a girdle or thong, something like a baby's nappy or diaper. In the eleventh century a quite different garment, similar to the trews or trousers of earlier times, was general. After that workmen again reverted to the shorter drawers and added hose (stockings) to cover the legs.

While the town-based artisan slowly began to assume a separate identity from the agricultural worker, the nobility became more concerned with maintaining their position and laws were enacted laying down what people might and might not wear. Charlemagne, for instance, decreed that peasants might only use coarse fabrics in dull

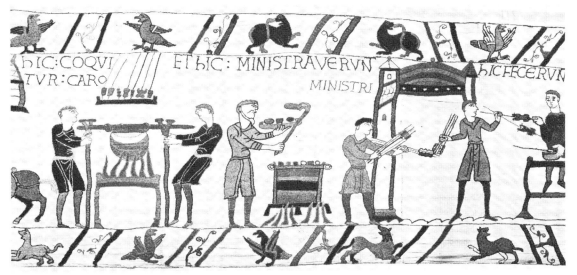

colours and had to keep their hair short, cut in a line with the middle of the forehead.

Throughout Europe from about A.D. 500 until the middle of the eleventh century there was little alteration in the knee-length tunic of the working man. Sleeves did get rather longer, possibly to allow them to be pulled over the hands for warmth, but also to enable them to be worn wrinkled and thus give greater freedom of movement. Neck openings were sometimes round and large enough to accommodate the head, but they might also be square, or split in front with the edges held together. (*Plate 1, fig. 5.*)

Some occupations were found to be easier to carry out when wearing little or nothing, and both sailors and miners often went naked. Sailors' clothes varied according to status and activity, those who climbed the rigging wore nothing, but steersmen needed cloaks and close-fitting caps.

The garments of country folk were heavier and rougher than those worn in towns and in England in the eleventh century shoe-wrights made special leather covers for the ankles of agricultural workers. Similar gaiters, or leggings, were to remain in use until the advent of the rubber boot.

Women continued to wear two tunics; by the eleventh century the underneath one showed at wrist and hem. The girdle was made of the same fabric as the overtunic. They kept their heads wrapped in a cloth or kerchief and, though occasionally barefoot, usually wore stockings and shoes of cloth.

Both men and women wore cloaks of coarse, rough wool which doubled as blankets; until the Norman Conquest hoods seem to have been more common on mainland Europe than in England.

Clothes were made in the wearers' homes or by serfs on big estates,

Norman cooks in belted tunics with long sleeves, depicted in the Bayeux Tapestry. (Late 11th century.)

though some early clothing factories probably came about through serfs producing more clothes than were required. In Anglo-Saxon England free labourers, a class who were not serfs but who had no land of their own, were supplied by their employers with shoes and gloves.

The colour of working clothes continued to be dull and those of serfs were usually of russet or grey. Sometimes, however, the retainers of the great families would use a colour that had been especially chosen, originally to be able to tell friend from foe in battle. These distinctive family colours led the way to heraldic motifs and then to livery, or uniform. Upper servants, such as stewards, were usually members of other noble families and dressed similarly to their employers. They could, however, be distinguished from them: it was usual for the nobility to wear hats indoors, therefore servants were not permitted to wear anything on their heads when actually in attendance.

Among the migrating races of the Dark Ages were the Normans. This vigorous and practical people, who seem to have been exceptionally good organisers, conquered a considerable part of Europe during the eleventh century. When they reached the Mediterranean countries they found cultures more advanced and more skilled than their own. Many of these skills they carried back with them to France and thence to England in 1066.

Although the conquerors' methods of manufacture and style of dress were better than their own, the Anglo-Saxon working people altered their clothing very little. However, the continental hooded cloak became general and remained an integral part of labouring dress throughout the Middle Ages, and a rural garment until comparatively modern times.

The dress of the lower classes throughout Europe changed hardly at all during the eleventh century, although the increasing splendour required by the nobility meant an improvement in the status of the artisan. Now quite distinct from the agricultural labourer, the town-dwelling artisan was assuming a higher position in the social ladder and beginning to make an effort to follow the fashion of the day.

The hooded cloak. Worn since ancient times.

2 Aprons and artisans

Medieval workers and specialist trades

WESTERN EUROPE EMERGED SLOWLY from the period commonly known as the Dark Ages and, although feudalism lingered, the fresh breezes of learning and religious revival began to blow away some of the worst excesses of serfdom. Two very different influences, coming from opposite directions, speeded up the change. The Crusades in their attempts to rescue the Holy Places from the 'infidel' brought the West into contact with Eastern culture, while the Plague, sweeping across Europe from Asia, had an even greater effect upon the lives of working people.

It has been estimated that in England alone the Plague carried off something like half the population, while its toll in the rest of Europe was equally devastating. Thriving on squalor and poverty, it decimated the work force, causing a scarcity of labour which eventually led to higher wages and the gradual erosion of the feudal system.

The Crusades, on the other hand, brought about improvements in trade and communications introducing an even more luxurious life-style for the wealthy. The spread of Eastern taste had far-reaching effects upon fashionable dress but little on the clothes of the peasant. However, the introduction of new fabrics and methods, along with a general increase in trade, meant that technical skills began to improve, giving the artisan and the tradesman far greater importance in the community.

In the later Middle Ages these specialists, ordinary peasants who had decided to concentrate on a particular craft, moved from the rural areas and, prospering in the growing towns, were able to dress better than the labourers they had left behind.

Centres of population remained widely scattered, although the Medieval castle, abbey, and manor housed large numbers of people and welcomed many travellers. The great majority of people, nevertheless, still only came into contact with those in their immediate neighbourhood and, if they did travel further afield, often had difficulty in making themselves understood. Even folk from adjoining parts of the same country sometimes had very different dialects.

Apart from the courts of rulers and noblemen, the meeting places were the fairs, ranging from the great cloth fairs of London and Bruges to the simple fairs of the country towns. The labour exchanges of the time, these fairs were also centres of trade and communication. News and goods otherwise only moved through the countryside with pedlar

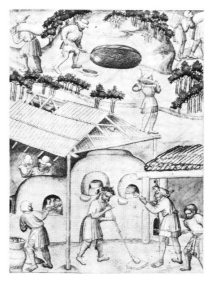

Glass-workers. The central figure is wearing only an under-tunic. (Early 15th-century manuscript)

and packhorse, the almost non-existent roads making progress slow and dangerous. Isolation like this required people to be self-sufficient in a way almost beyond our modern comprehension and it accounts to a great extent for the lack of change in the dress of rural and agricultural workers.

The manufacture of clothing continued to be a major preoccupation of rural people and much of it was done by women while the men worked in the fields. The spinning wheel made its appearance in the twelfth century and young girls were so often engaged in using it that in England 'spinster' came to denote an unmarried woman. The clothes they made were mostly of coarse wool (home-spun, home-dyed and hand-woven), of coarse unbleached linen, resembling what is now called canvas or burlap, and, in the southern parts of Europe, of cotton. Garments had to last for years—many must have passed from one generation to another—for technical skills were limited and, although looms were improving, scissors and needles were scarce.

It is hardly surprising, therefore, that working dress varied little from occupation to occupation and from century to century. Nevertheless, in spite of the poverty and the conditions under which both serf and freeman lived, contemporary accounts suggest that by the start of the fourteenth century the English worker at least was warmly clad in 'body linen, woollen garments and shoes'.

Body linen, or what is now known as underwear, was for men short linen drawers or a simple loincloth pulled between the legs. Decency had to be maintained as best it could and poverty was no excuse; the absence of the undergarment was considered shameful even when the tunic covered the discrepancy. The Franciscan Order, founded in the thirteenth century, adopted the very basic garments of the poorest Italian worker, drawers, tunic and girdle.

Most people wore two tunics and women sometimes added an undergarment as well. Worn in its simplest form, two rectangles of linen with shoulder straps, by the bath attendants of Prague, this chemise was for a time an occupational costume in its own right. (*Plate 3, fig. 12.*)

Though possessions were few, some, like knives and purses hung from belt or girdle, can sometimes help to indicate the occupations of the many working people who appear in illuminated manuscripts.

Although the exquisite colours in these manuscripts must be treated with caution, their brilliant hues, possibly depicting an artistic and ideal life rather than a realistic one, do show that there was considerable variation in the colour and use of the basic garments. 'Hodden' (natural, or unbleached) grey, and red-brown, or russet—the name of a fabric, as well as a colour—were common among working people, but blue, green, and orange were also widely used; all these being dyes readily available from common plants. National variations meant that in the Netherlands, Flanders, and parts of France, dull red was much worn because the madder from which it came was widespread. In Ireland saffron yellow, either from the winter crocus or other vegetable sources, was popular until forbidden for political reasons.

The sumptuary, or expenditure, laws in Ireland were unusual in that they were political. Elsewhere, although often ineffective in spite of their number, the laws were an attempt to strengthen privilege and prevent people being extravagant. In most sumptuary laws of the Middle Ages it was fabric and decoration that were the issue, which meant that they had a certain influence upon occupational dress. In England in the middle of the fourteenth century, for instance, tradesmen and artisans were forbidden to wear expensive cloth, while labourers and servants had to use fabric that cost even less.

There were also restrictions on the types of fur people might use. Many garments were lined with it as it was vital for warmth, both indoors and out, but working people had to be content with the domestic animals like cat, dog and sheep, or the smaller wild ones like badger and fox.

In the eleventh century trousers or breeches had come to the ankles and were often wound round with strips of material like bandages, or worn with cloth hose roughly cut to the shape of the leg. They gradually shrank, however, to thigh length where the hose rose to meet them—the trousers eventually became merely underwear. They were covered completely when the hose were joined to each other to form a garment like modern tights and kept in place by being attached to the undertunic with ties.

These hose were sometimes without feet, but until the late fourteenth century not as a rule close-fitting. However, when they did fit tightly and had to be worn for jobs that required bending or kneeling,

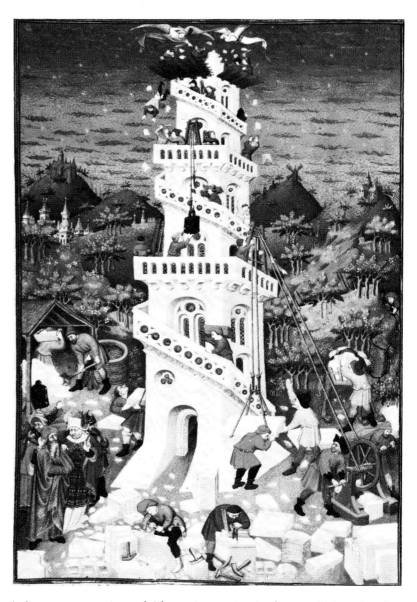

Builders in a variety of working clothes. (15th-century manuscript)

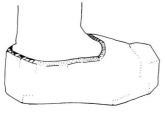

Medieval wooden shoe.

holes were sometimes deliberately cut in the knees. Although soles could be attached to the hose, working people generally needed the protection of leather footwear, while shoes made of wood and others with wooden soles were useful for keeping out the wet.

Both sexes wore head-coverings at all times, irrespective of class or occupation.

Although the basic clothes of the poorer sections of the community changed slowly between 1100 and 1300, the upper tunic took a number of different forms. By the mid-fourteenth century it usually fitted fairly closely but it could either be fastened in front or put on over the head, as had been the case earlier.

Agricultural workers' clothes have always needed to be warm in winter, cool in summer and permit ease of movement. In the Middle Ages hooded capes were often used as they allowed freedom of the arms, while providing protection for head and shoulders. Serving the same function when combined with separate hoods were various over-garments. One of these, shaped like a modern poncho and worn in the fourteenth century, may well have been the forerunner of that most famous rural garment—the smock. Ploughmen in one beautiful manuscript are shown warmly dressed in these ponchos, or tabards, with hoods and hats. On their legs they wear cloth hose, and boots bound round the leg with laces passing through slots. On their hands are gloves or mittens with several compartments. (*Plate 2, fig. 10.*) Hand-coverings of this kind, though popular in England at the time, are seldom to be seen on women, possibly because they did not do much field work in winter.

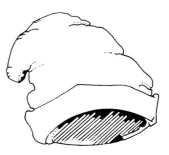

Close-fitting cap. Worn since ancient times.

In many parts of Europe men are shown in warm weather as wearing merely the long trousers (*Plate 2, fig. 7*), or the shorter drawers, with or without undertunic or shirt. They are also shown working for coolness and comfort in the shirt alone. Barefooted women looped up their overskirts and put straw hats over their kerchiefs when at work in the hay fields. Straw hats, or hats made of lime bark, were worn in most countries although the shapes varied, some had distinct crowns and wide brims while others were of a coolie style. (*Plate 3, fig. 13.*) Only peasants and travellers wore brimmed hats.

Probably the most easily recognizable occupation in early Medieval times was that of the shepherd who, because of his religious significance, is often to be seen in contemporary illustrations and sculptures. They were also, of course, important because the economy of a number of countries was dependent upon sheep. In England by the fifteenth century there were about three sheep to every human being. Almost invariably shepherds were well and warmly dressed in wool, with tunics often longer than those of other rural people. In winter hooded tunics or cloaks (*Plate 2, fig. 6*) were frequently of either sheep or goatskin, with the fur on the outside, and worn with leg bandages. Wide felt hats were used to keep off sun and rain.

Besides strips of fabric, labourers also wound wisps of straw round their legs as a protection not only from cold but also from thorns and stubble. The better-off had gaiters or leggings of leather. Other forms of protective clothing were not unknown. Bee-veils were used to protect the face when working at the hives and at least one contemporary illustration shows a metal worker in goggles.

Apart from additions for protection or convenience, basic working clothes varied little from one occupation to another. Although they sometimes indicate the type of work which a man is engaged upon, it is hard to decide when such additions are clothes and when tools. Of this

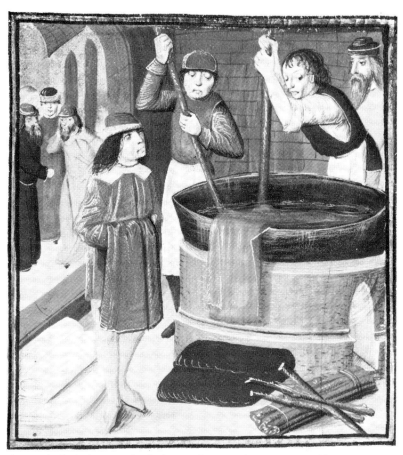

Flemish dyers at work
wearing aprons.
(Manuscript c.1482)

the seed-cloth is a particularly good example. In the Middle Ages this rectangle of linen was knotted behind the neck and, when the other two ends were held in one hand, it formed a pouch from which seed was thrown broadcast. (*Plate 5, fig. 21.*)

Something like the seed- or sowing-cloth, and also used for carrying, was the apron which, more than any other garment, has persisted as a part of working dress. Although it has sometimes been used as a tool, its most important aspect is the protection it offers to the worker and to his or her clothes.

Damage to the body and to the clothing is usually the result of the work the hands are doing in front of the body. Preventing damage to the person is part of the instinct of self-preservation; protection of the clothes is also important for those to whom they are essential for warmth and decency but who cannot afford to be continually replacing them. The apron, therefore, has always played a very important part in working dress and has frequently been adapted to suit a particular occupation.

An ancient form of apron is the leather one worn by blacksmiths and farriers who need protection from the hooves of the horses they are shoeing and from the heat and sparks of the forge. In Medieval times the shape of this apron was often irregular as it was made from a whole skin to cover as much of the body as possible. It was either pinned on the chest or held with a loop around the neck.

Most aprons of the period, however, were without bibs. In the most basic form, such as that worn by cooks, it was no more than a rough cloth. Craftsmen and artisans wore short aprons gathered in a band that tied around the waist, while similar but longer versions were worn by butchers and others who had particularly messy work to do. (*Plate 3, fig. 14.*)

The fact that the apron in the Middle Ages was added by men specifically for work is borne out in a number of Medieval manuscripts where Christ is shown as wearing an apron while washing the feet of his disciples.

Aprons with bibs were rare at this period but a woman blacksmith (there were female wheelwrights, brewers and shoemakers, too!) is shown wearing one that is looped round the neck. (*Plate 3, fig. 11.*)

Usually of hemp or linen, most aprons in England and France were white, though in some other countries colours were more common. On English women's aprons, honeycombing, an early form of smocking, was sometimes used to gather the fabric into the waistband. (*Plate 2, fig. 9.*)

Working women's dress generally consisted of a long-sleeved under-tunic and a shorter-sleeved, or sleeveless, overtunic. (*Plate 2, fig. 9.*) On the head was a white kerchief or hood, either hanging loose or wrapped round under the chin. Hair nets with a caul, an arrangement of bands to keep the net in place, were also used. (*Plate 3, fig. 11.*)

Some colour distinctions now existed between occupations. Millers usually dressed in white, not for reasons of hygiene but because if they had worn other colours they would always have looked as though they had been dipped in flour. Foresters, on the other hand, wore green as a camouflage.

Towards the end of the fifteenth century men began to work in the short undertunic or doublet to which, for some time, the hose had been attached by means of ties. As these hose now fitted more closely, it was necessary for the ties or 'points' to be undone during strenuous activity. (*Plate 3, fig. 15.*)

Some women worked in the great households of the time though not, as might have been expected, as cooks, for this was to remain an exclusively male occupation for some time to come. Apart from the apron, women household servants wore no special form of clothing.

Male servants, potential fighting men, were exceedingly numerous. Hordes of them accompanied noblemen wherever they went to add to their dignity and status. By the middle of the fourteenth century they were dressed in livery. This term had originally referred to all payments in kind, including food, but it now described the particular type or colour of dress worn by men-servants. As such, it can probably be called the first uniform. Livery usually bore insignia of some kind, with a crest or coat or arms which, when out of livery, the servant wore on his ordinary dress.

Ostentation in the clothes of servants was a way of displaying wealth and eventually became so widespread that a number of laws were made to curb what has since been called 'conspicuous consumption'—the deliberate display of finery in order to impress.

The more important positions in the great households were still generally held by noblemen who dressed in the fashion of the day but, as before, they uncovered their heads when actually in attendance.

Aprons, though later to indicate domestic occupations, were worn by few servants apart from cooks and those actually engaged in the serving of food and drink. Even then, the apron was not always used but the waiter's napkin, or cloth, placed over shoulder or arm, was already traditional.

Throughout Medieval times the herald was an important member of noble households and wore a particular style of dress. This was a tabard consisting of two rectangles joined over the shoulders and reaching to the knees or just above but, unlike the tunic, without belt or girdle. Two further panels were attached, one above each shoulder to form a sort of open sleeve. On the front of the tabard the herald carried the insignia or cognisance of his master.

An allowance of clothes was part of a servant's wage and royal retainers received wearing apparel twice a year—a set for summer and a set for winter. Among royal servants were the first official London watchmen appointed in 1253 who, as they wore the king's insignia, might be considered the first public servants. As well as his badge the king gave them *strawen* hats, although the usual function of straw hats as a protection from the sun can hardly have been the reason for their use.

From the twelfth century the spread of learning gradually led to the growth of the professions as educated laymen began to take over some of the functions previously performed by the Church. They adopted a quasi-religious style of dress and, when the fashionable world began to wear the 'short' costume in the middle of the fifteenth century, they still retained the long *houppelande*, or gown. The robes worn today by judges and barristers in England, as well as in many other parts of the world, and robes used by academic and civil dignitaries, are descended from these, continuing the idea that dignity, learning and authority are best indicated by extra long and archaic garments. Though occasionally black, the gowns of the professions were usually of bright colours and rich fabrics, frequently trimmed with the rarer furs. These imposing garments were to be seen throughout Europe: an Italian magistrate wore scarlet velvet trimmed with fur, while a German judge dressed in brocaded velvet.

For a long time medicine had been the prerogative of the Church, but in 1163 the Pope forbade monks to practise surgery and the medical profession began to take shape. Physicians wore the long gown and a distinctive cap (*Plate 2, fig. 8*), although surgeons, being considered surgical workmen rather than academics, were entitled to neither; nor were they allowed the coif, a black or white linen cap that fitted the head and covered the ears.

Out of doors a mantle, or long, hooded cloak, was worn over the long gown by professional men, but this was also forbidden to surgeons and to the lesser members of other professions, such as notaries or clerks.

However, in spite of their efforts, the professions did not succeed in restricting the long gown to their own use as, by the end of the fifteenth century, the increased prosperity of merchants and master craftsmen meant that it was worn by them as well as by bankers, architects and master builders.

3 Sumptuary laws and livery

The sixteenth century

PERHAPS THE BEST DESCRIPTION of the sixteenth century is contained in one word—expansive. As the period following the Renaissance it was only natural that the new age, like a new infant, should show its healthy growth in this way.

Learning, trade, prosperity and clothes all expanded. It is only necessary to look at pictures of the great rulers of the period, Henry VIII and Elizabeth I of England, or Charles V of France, to see how much actual space this physical expansion needed. Clothes and ideas were bursting out all over.

To grow, either physically or spiritually, a certain amount of freedom is required which the gradual disappearance of feudalism was providing and, as the process was faster in England than in either France or Germany, her rural population was the most prosperous of the three. By the middle of the century the Renaissance was at its height in England and there, as elsewhere, religious beliefs were changing. However, in spite of this, and in spite of religious wars in France and the Inquisition in Spain, trade between Europe and the Far East and India increased. Improvements in shipbuilding and navigation led to more exploration and to the greatest expansion of all, colonization.

In England increasing trade, with the consequent greater importance of merchants and bankers, meant the main centres of population grew. London, unlike many cities on the European continent, still managed to keep one foot in the countryside. This was possibly due to the fact that many of the young men apprenticed to merchants and craftsmen were the sons of landowners and maintained their links with home.

A further link between town and country in England was due to the growth of the cloth trade and the way in which, to satisfy the needs of customers with an ever-improving standard of living, merchants began to involve more and more rural people in cloth production. From merely distributing the raw materials, merchants now began to supply the manufacturing equipment that had previously been jealously held on to by the towns. As a result, the number of manufactories increased and the cloth trade grew so large that it became, and remained, second in importance to agriculture for centuries.

The expansion of the cloth trade led to many changes in English rural life, not the least of which was the enclosure of land for the raising of sheep—land that had previously employed many labourers in the growing of crops. Together with the breaking up of the great monasteries by Henry VIII this resulted in much unemployment and hardship.

Some of those who had lost their occupation through the changes obtained work as servants with the new owners of the monastery lands. The number of retainers continued to increase and great nobles travelled from one place to another with two or three hundred men in livery. Worn by all but the most exalted and the most menial servants, livery was so often blue that this colour came to be thought of as the mark of servility and avoided by other members of society.

The clothes of ordinary people were broadly similar to those of the more prosperous but made of simpler, coarser fabrics and with less decoration. Amongst rural women the major change at this period was the separation of the bodice from the skirt. When the weather became warm, or the latest addition to the family had to be fed, it was easier to remove a bodice from over the chemise than to take off the complete gown or tunic. Although the growing clothes-consciousness of towns-people was beginning to be felt by country folk, they were still mainly concerned with more practical matters.

The banded skirt, which eventually became an integral part of rural dress, made its appearance about this time. Starting off as an urban garment, its possibilities were soon realised by thrifty country women. A fabric band round the hem of a skirt increased durability, while bands added higher up could either hide a pleat made when shortening a garment made for someone else, or hide the place where such a pleat had been removed.

The apron was now universally worn in Europe and with kerchief, hat, chemise, gown, or bodice and skirt, it formed the dress of the rural working woman that was to remain, with only slight modifications, for centuries.

In men's costume the major change was the introduction of the jerkin or coat that could be either sleeved (*Plate 6, fig. 28*) or sleeveless. Tunics continued to be used however, particularly in the country and by servants: they were worn belted and with hose and shoes, or calf-length boots. For the extra warmth and protection he needed a shepherd might wear two very much longer tunics. (*Plate 4, fig. 18.*) The new jerkin was frequently removed for work to show what was now a shirt and, invariably, white. Short breeches appeared towards the middle of the period and were worn by some craftsmen with shirt and apron. (*Plate 5, fig. 25.*)

Ill-fitting hose were less seen now as fabric had more elasticity and could be better tailored for a closer fit. Convenience and warmth, the first two requirements of working dress, may have been satisfied by these 'tights' but where the tunic had been replaced by the short jerkin

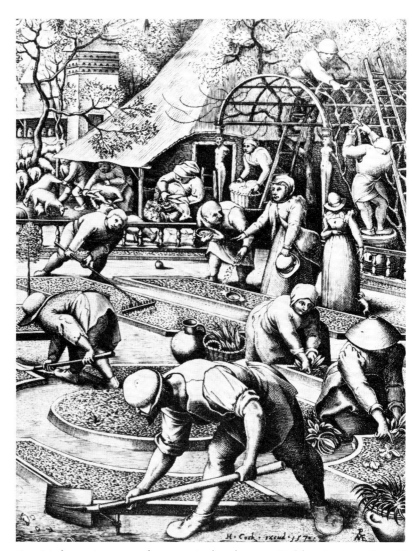

Dutch gardeners. Some of the men are in sleeveless jerkins. (Engraving by Petrus à Mercia [1590] from a painting by Pieter van der Heyden)

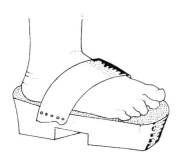

16th-century sandal.

the third requirement, decency, had to be supplied by the insertion of what was known as a codpiece. (This separate covering of the fly-opening was the very reverse of decent when worn in its exaggerated padded form by men of fashion.) Labourers would have found this type of codpiece inconvenient even if it had not been, as was the case in some countries, forbidden them by law. Hose were sometimes made without heels or toes, being held in place by a band under the instep (*Plate 4, fig. 17*), probably a utilitarian device to make them last longer by avoiding the hole-rubbing action of coarse or ill-fitting shoes. Occasionally they were completely footless and dagged (roughly cut) round the ankle to prevent fraying.

Cloth and leather leggings or gaiters, used on their own in summer as a protection against stubble, and over hose in winter for warmth, were worn by many countrymen.

Women's bodices varied, a front- or back-lacing sleeveless corset-bodice being more common on the European continent than in England. The bodice was often removed for harvesting and similar work, the chemise being used on its own with apron and skirt bunched up for ease of movement. (*Plate 5, fig. 22.*) Where the gown was still used it was long-sleeved and worn with an apron and a white kerchief. (*Plate 4, fig. 16.*) When the skirt, whether separate or part of a gown, was looped up for convenience the undergarment, as it was shorter, retained its normal length. A brushed or 'thrummed' felt hat was worn over the kerchief when the weather was unsuitable for straw.

Unlike men servants, most of whom wore livery, women servants had no particular style of dress and this was partly because most of their work was done out of sight of anyone whom their employers might wish to impress. Although it may seem unfair that they did not receive an allowance of clothes twice a year like their male counterparts, they might as a result be more fashionably dressed, for the mistress of the house and her daughters traditionally passed, or 'cast', their clothes to them. Even where this did not occur the women tended to be influenced by urban fashion, which was itself a version of fashionable dress. In some places, parts of Germany for instance, women servants wore no shoes indoors, although this seems to have been unusual elsewhere. Skirts were rather shorter than was fashionable, and various types of apron were worn according to the kind of work to be done. A maid-servant in Wales about the year 1600 had three, one of linen, one of flannel, and one of black cloth.

It is certain that both male and female servants attempted to follow fashion and their masters sometimes provided very elaborate clothes for them. This is evident from the number of sumptuary laws in which they are mentioned. One law in the reign of Henry VIII permitted them no more than 'three broad yards' for gown or coat, and forbade the use of any fur but lambskin. By the time of Elizabeth the gown was rather old-fashioned but was still worn by servants in winter, although, to prevent confusion with the professional classes who also retained it, it had to be calf-length. A pleasantly humane touch about this law was that it permitted the gown to be longer if the servant was very old!

The use of the 'buff', or leather jerkin, by men servants at this period may possibly, as it had originally been a military garment, have signified that a master still had the right to call upon his servants to fight for him.

When trunk-hose were fashionable in the middle of the century servants were not allowed to use much padding. Among the servants who did not wear livery were cooks who added aprons to ordinary working dress of jerkin and hose; a long cloth like that used by waiters was sometimes worn around the neck and protected the hands when hot utensils had to be moved. (*Plate 5, fig. 24.*)

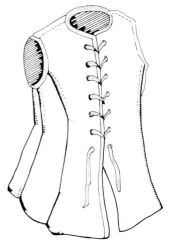

16th-century leather jerkin.

Besides being much worn by servants, blue was the colour considered suitable for those who served the community, such as beadles (the sixteenth-century equivalent of policemen), and also for apprentices who were in a master/servant relationship while serving their time in a trade. Their blue coats, white breeches and yellow stockings amounted to a uniform and were a common sight in the streets for many years. (*Plate 6, fig. 30.*) Although often the sons of wealthy men, apprentices had their behaviour and their clothing rigorously controlled. Flogging was one of the means used and the administrator of this punishment wore a particular garment to preserve his anonymity. Made like a sack, it had eye-holes and arm-holes. The floggings must have been severe as the mere sight of the dress was often sufficient to scare a sinner into submission. Known as a 'bulbeggar', this symbol of retribution gave rise to a threat that, even in the present century, was used to frighten children—'the bogeyman will get you'!

A flat, round hat that appeared early in the century 'couched fast to the pate like an oyster' (oysters were a plentiful and comparatively cheap food at the time) eventually became the everyday wear of apprentices and citizens, becoming known as the 'city flat cap'. For about twenty-five years at the end of the century, in an attempt to protect the English wool trade, the law required that woollen caps be worn—except on Sundays and holy days—by all who were not of noble rank. As a result, the flat cap was also the workday wear of artisans and labourers.

The use of the apron for protection was now widespread. Blacksmiths, farriers and shoemakers used leather ones, often a whole skin held by a button or a pin to the jacket, or by a thong round the neck. Coarse, white bibless aprons were still worn by most artisans, men serving at table, brewers, butchers (*Plate 6, fig. 29*), and others handling foodstuffs, while farm labourers continued to use seed-cloths when sowing grain. As the law enforcing woollen caps shows, there was quite a distinction between working dress and Sunday clothes: a tradesman might be called to task by his fellows if he wore working clothes on high days and holidays. He was also liable to be fined, as a butcher was when he wore a coat of *freize* (coarse woollen cloth) when attending a meeting of his livery company. These trade associations were so-called not because the members wore servants' livery, or a particular kind of occupational dress, but because when they met they had to wear a specified gown or other formal garment that befitted their position as masters of their 'art, mysterie and manual occupation'.

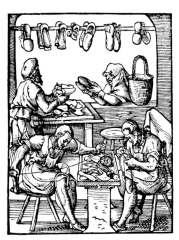

Shoemakers at work in bibbed aprons.
(Jost Amman and Hans Sachs *The Book of Trades,* 1568)

A type of apron that clearly indicated a particular job was the bibless check one English barbers wore until the seventeenth century; so unique were these that barbers were often called 'checkered apron men'. Another distinctive apron was worn by central European miners; this, unlike most aprons, protected the back because, when working in a

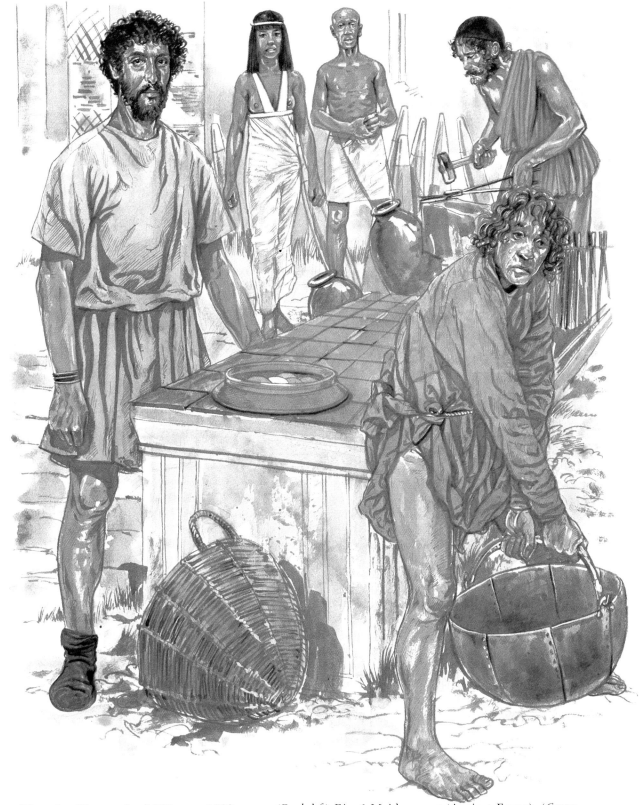

Plate 1 Chapter 1—3000 B.C.-1100 A.D. (*Back left*) *Fig. 1* Maid-servant (Ancient Egypt), (*Centre back*) *Fig. 2* Workman (Ancient Egypt), (*Back right*) *Fig. 3* Blacksmith (Ancient Greece), (*Front left*) *Fig. 4* Butcher (Roman), (*Front right*) *Fig. 5* Labourer (Norman Britain).

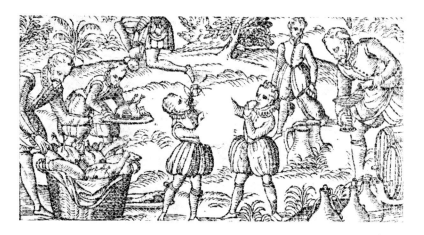

Servants at a royal picnic. The butler (right) is wearing a small apron. (Engraving from G. Turberville, *Noble Art of Venerie*, 1575?)

stooping position, it is more vulnerable than the front. Made of leather, these also provided the miner with something waterproof to sit on when he needed it. Not all miners of the time wore special clothing, for those doing open-cast work in Spain are shown in ordinary working dress. (*Plate 6, fig. 26.*) An English miner of about 1570, although wearing fashionable breeches under a belted tunic, carried a candle in his mouth and wore an unusual oval cap that may possibly have been padded.

Two trades that tended to be more fashionably dressed than others were masons and tailors. Masons, who held a position of some importance in the community, protected their clothes with an apron but the tailor did not. A tailor could only be recognized for what he was if he happened to carry one of his threaded needles in his coat or if, like one famous clothier, he used his codpiece as a pincushion.

With exploration and the expansion of trade, sailors had become more important and were developing a style of dress of their own, adopting and adapting garments that had already been found convenient. Trousers had been known from pre-Roman times and had never entirely disappeared; worn by fishermen in various countries including the Netherlands and the Basque region of Spain, they had now become traditional for most seafarers, as well as for inland watermen like the Venetian gondoliers. Long and full, the trousers were made of coarse fabric, or even sailcloth, and were wide enough to be rolled up for work on board. Sleeveless leather jerkins were also worn by sailors over their shirts (*Plate 4, fig. 18*), and by the end of the century many had high, shaggy hats of fur or felt which fitted closely to the head. Fishermen, though not as a rule sailors, also used leather leggings.

Landsmen in coastal areas used trousers, too, although they did not roll them up but tied them below the knee, a practice that was to continue for centuries wherever they were adopted for labouring work.

One result of overseas expansion and colonization was an increase in the number and variety of furs from the New World. In some places

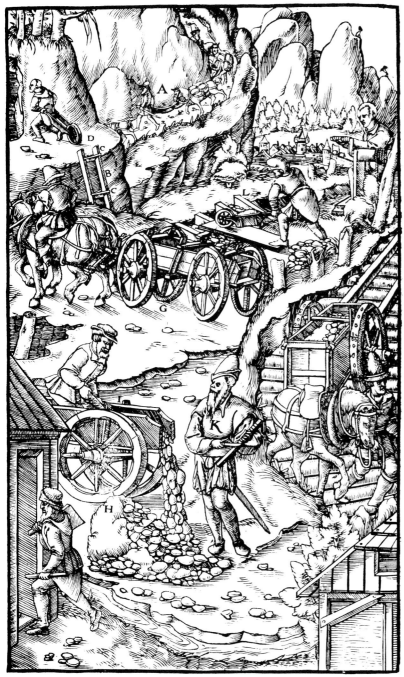

Mine workers. Some are wearing the protective back apron. (*Agricole De re Metallica*, 1561)

these were used as a form of currency and those who carried on the trade, the merchants, lost no opportunity of advertising their wares by using them. So widespread did this become that a fur-trimmed gown was the accepted costume of a merchant.

Fur also trimmed and lined the gowns of architects, aldermen, scholars, lawyers and physicians as well as those of 'elder statesmen'.

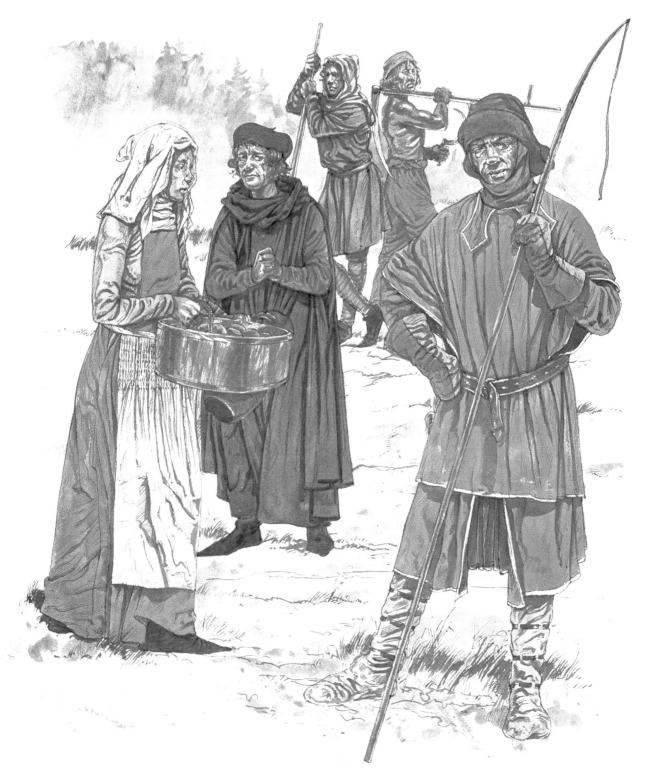

Plate 2 Chapter 2—12th-14th century (*Back left*) *Fig.* 6 Shepherd (England 12th century), (*Back right*) *Fig.* 7 Labourer (France 13th century), (*Centre*) *Fig.* 8 Physician (France late 13th century), (*Front left*) *Fig.* 9 Rural worker (England early 14th century), (*Front right*) *Fig. 10* Ploughman (England early 14th century).

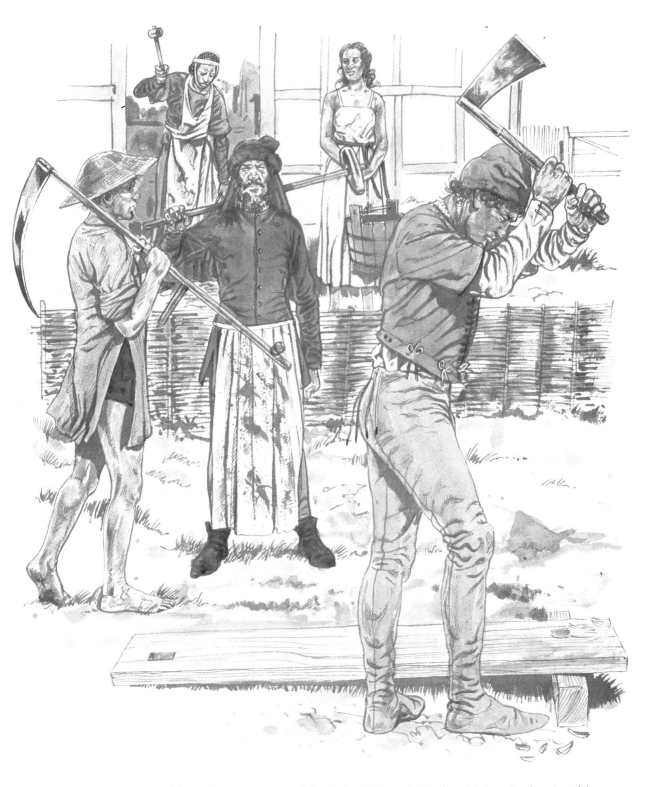

Plate 3   Chapter 2—14th-15th century   (*Back left*) *Fig. 11* Female blacksmith (England early 14th century), (*Back right*) *Fig. 12* Bath attendant (Bohemia late 14th century), (*Front left*) *Fig. 13* Harvester (France early 15th century), (*Centre Front*) *Fig. 14* Butcher (France 15th century), (*Front right*) *Fig. 15* Carpenter (France 15th century).

The combination of the out-of-date garment with costly fur and fabric must have been particularly impressive at a time when men of fashion were wearing short, bulky clothes.

As well as the gown, professional men, though not merchants, still wore the linen coif of either black or white. (*Plate 6, fig. 27.*)

Medicine was still largely under the influence of the Church and a rather ecclesiastical appearance was to be seen in the dress of those connected with it. A surgeon from the Netherlands in 1569, for instance, wore a white habit with a cap and cowl. Up to 1546 most nursing had been done by nuns, and even when the hospitals were secularized those who worked in them tended to have the appearance of members of a religious order, special cloth being provided for their 'habits' at regular intervals. About the middle of the century blue was adopted and most nurses have worn this colour from that time until the recent arrival of the white overall. Nurses' head-dresses tended to be those of their particular area and period, though usually white.

It is possible that the medical profession was the first to have specific regulations laid down for protective clothing as, in 1555, English students of anatomy had to provide their lecturers with two white shoulder-high aprons and two pairs of oversleeves. Other protective garments during the sixteenth century were bee-veils for apiarists in Italy, goggles for metal workers in France, and gloves for reapers in England; in Spain a carefully arranged kerchief protected women cleaning corn from inhaling the dust as they worked. (*Plate 4, fig. 20.*)

4   Sombre ideas and sober clothes

Work and religion in the seventeenth century

THE SEVENTEENTH CENTURY was a time of rearrangement and change in Europe and the democratic ideas that were emerging inevitably had their effect upon the clothes of the period. It is hardly surprising, therefore, that by the end of the era working dress had many of the attributes familiar in the twentieth century.

In an age of contrasts there was tremendous luxury and tremendous poverty, but the differences in dress between one end of the spectrum and the other was largely the difference between what was essential and what was excessive. However, in spite of the Puritan influences of the time, the rapidly increasing prosperity of merchant and tradesman made the nobility more determined than ever to keep the gap between the classes wide. Frequent changes of fashion attempted to achieve this for communications had improved to such an extent that the town dweller was able to copy the dress of the nobility much more quickly than before. But, human nature being what it is, not even frequent fashion changes and sumptuary laws had the desired effect. It was, however, achieved for a while by religion.

This conflict between classes was an indication of the great conflicts of ideas and ideals. Extremes of all kinds existed, but it was the extremes of religious thought that led to confrontation, persecution and war.

The tendency towards the adoption of plain and sombre clothes, virtually the dress of well-to-do working people, was hastened and spread by the rule of the Cromwellian Government in England and by the persecution of the Protestants in France during the reign of Louis XIV. The deliberate avoidance of ostentation by the middle classes might today be called a 'gesture of solidarity' for it was the outward and visible sign of support for an ideal.

The French Protestants, many of whom were craftsmen and artisans, had been an important part of the French economy and when they were forced to leave their home country in their thousands they took many skills to the lands of their adoption. Settling chiefly in England, Ireland, Prussia, North America and the recently formed Dutch colony at the Cape of Good Hope, they added greatly to the prosperity of crafts and industries. Partly because of this, however, there began from now on to be an increasing gap between the tradesman or master craftsman and the labourer or unskilled worker.

From Medieval times guilds had existed for each trade and were

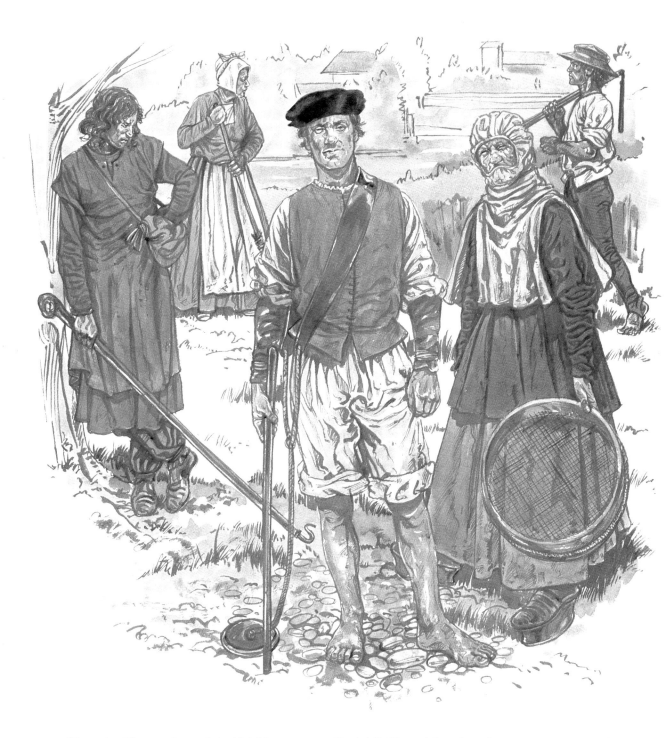

Plate 4 Chapter 3—early/mid 16th century (*Back left*) *Fig. 16* Rural worker (South Netherlands), (*Back right*) *Fig. 17* Rural worker (France), (*Front left*) *Fig. 18* Shepherd (Spain), (*Centre front*) *Fig. 19* Sailor (Spain), (*Front right*) *Fig. 20* Rural worker winnowing (Spain).

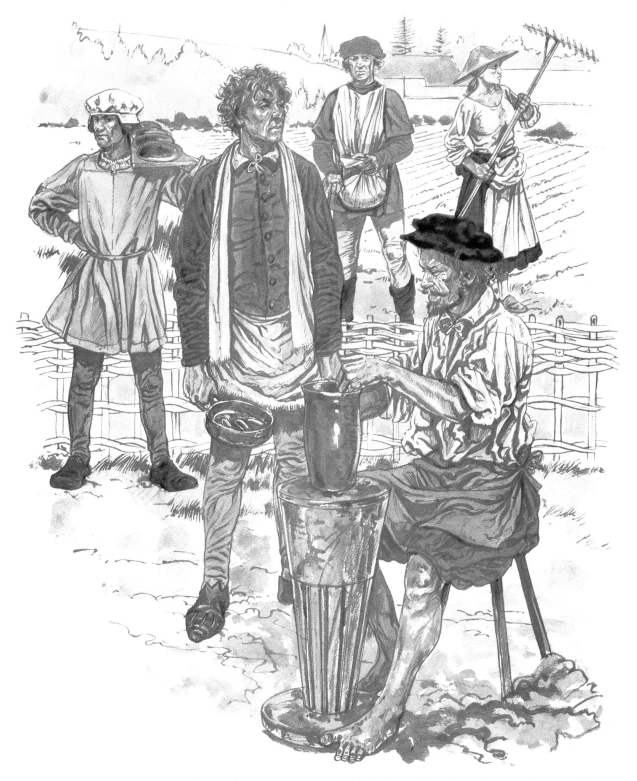

Plate 5 Chapter 3—early/mid 16th century (*Back left*) *Fig. 21* Rural worker, sowing (South Netherlands), (*Back right*) *Fig. 22* Rural worker, harvesting (Netherlands), (*Front left*) *Fig. 23* Baker (Netherlands), (*Centre front*) *Fig. 24* Cook (Germany), (*Front right*) *Fig. 25* Potter (Germany).

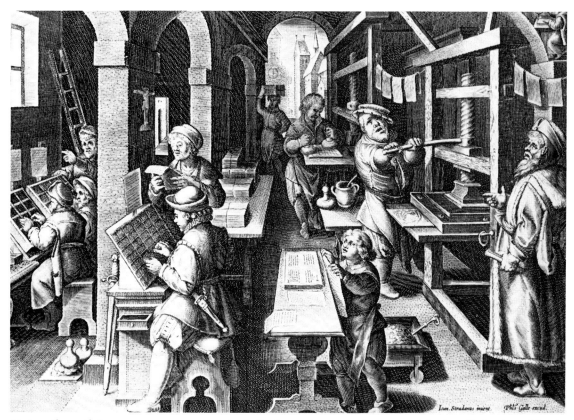

Only a few of the workers at this printing press wear aprons but nearly all have hats. (Stradanus c. 1600)

composed of all the various people engaged in it, all sharing alike in prosperity and in hardship. But things began to change as the distinctions between tradesman and labourer grew and differences in dress emphasized the split.

Another division that showed in dress was that between town and country. Although farmers and agricultural workers in England at the start of the century were very prosperous and wore clothes not very different from those of the well-to-do, townspeople in some countries were beginning to develop a style of dress of their own. National characteristics were also starting to emerge, but the basic working dress throughout Europe was similar and the changes only came about gradually.

The Medieval tunic had almost vanished although its place was soon to be taken by a somewhat similar garment, the smock. At the start of the period, however, most workmen wore shirts, jackets or jerkins, with breeches, wide felt hats, or the more convenient close-fitting caps. Women wore a bodice somewhat similar to the man's jerkin but with a chemise instead of a shirt; the chemise now had a much fuller sleeve and either a gathered neckline or a rolled collar. The overskirt was usually tucked up for work and showed the shorter, and somewhat coarse, underskirt beneath. The bibless apron was of various colours

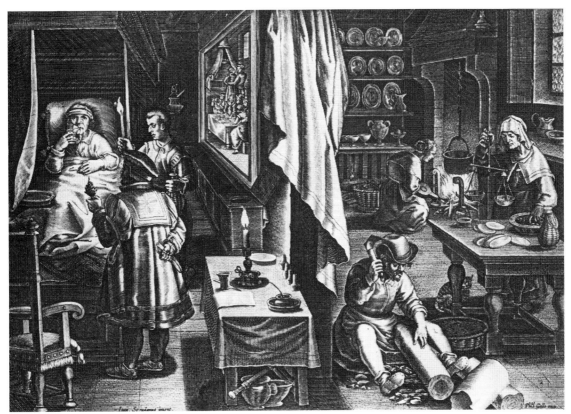

Doctor visiting a patient and servants at work in the kitchen. (Stradanus c.1600)

but the coif or head-dress, though it varied considerably in style, was always white. Out of doors it was covered with a straw or felt hat, but some women who had to carry weights on their heads wore head-pads as a protection and to balance the load. (*Plate 7, fig. 31.*)

The bodices and jerkins (also called jackets, coats, and waistcoats) could be either sleeved or sleeveless. Climate had something to do with this as at the start of the century the garments tended to have sleeves in England, Germany, northern France and the Netherlands, while in the warmer parts of Europe and in the colonies they were more likely to be without sleeves. Also, in the early years, the neckline of the women's bodice was square and fastened with hooks or laces, usually in front, but occasionally at the back.

Dull colours and black predominated, highlighted by white coif, collar, shirt and chemise. The use of grey was so widespread at this time that young French working girls were nick-named *grisettes*, a term that was to remain with them even though colour began to creep back into working dress towards the end of the century.

The all-over style, of course, was that which eventually became known as Puritan costume, combining as it did the basics of working dress—warmth, convenience and decency. These fundamental attributes were those required by the Puritans who also found in working

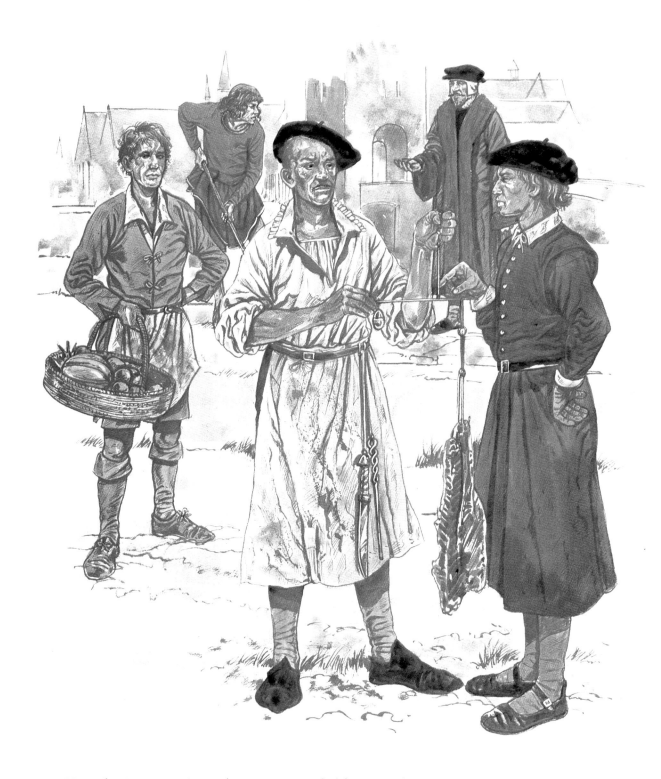

Plate 6 Chapter 3—late 16th century (*Back left*) *Fig. 26* Miner (*Spain*), (*Back right*) *Fig. 27* Physician (England), (*Front left*) *Fig. 28* Market porter (Italy), (*Centre front*) *Fig. 29* Butcher (Italy), (*Centre right*) *Fig. 30* Apprentice (England).

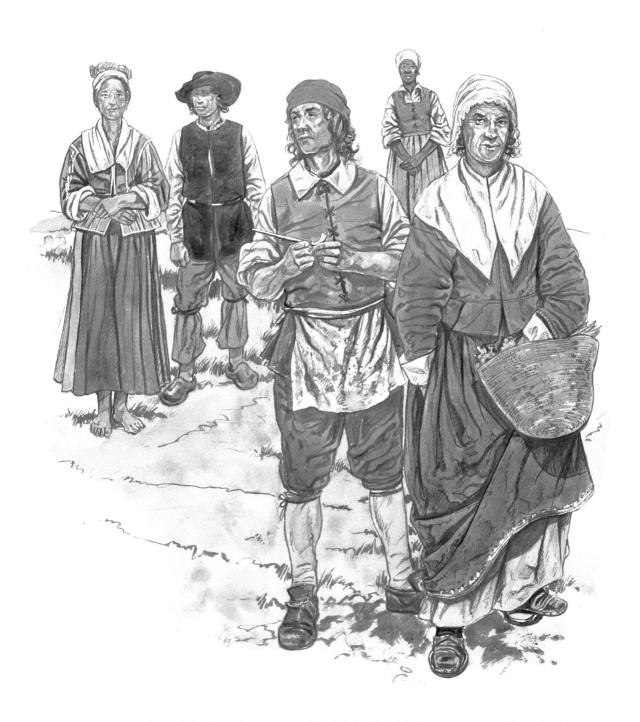

Plate 7 Chapter 4—early/mid 17th century (*Back left*) *Fig. 31* Countrywoman (France), (*Centre back*) *Fig. 32* Labourer (Netherlands), (*Centre right*) *Fig. 33* Maid-servant (Cape of Good Hope), (*Front left*) *Fig. 34* Printer (England), (*Front right*) *Fig. 35* Countrywoman (England).

dress a lack of display which accorded well with their beliefs. Particularly associated with them for a very long period was the large white kerchief that working women wore round their necks. (*Plates 7, 8, 9, figs 35, 40, 44.*) The starched ruff and its successor the high collar were never worn by workers on account of their discomfort.

Quite naturally there was, in all occupations, a lot of difference in dress between those who prospered and those who did not. At all periods the latter clothed themselves in the best assortment of rags available, and the seventeenth century was no exception. The difference between the well-off farmer and a poverty-stricken labourer was bound to be enormous. Generally speaking, however, in the countryside men dressed in fairly loose jerkins with shirt, baggy breeches, and woollen hose which had ceased to be tights and had become stockings again. At periods when the breeches were close-fitting the fastening below the knee was usually left open. Leather breeches were common, particularly in North America. More durable and weatherproof than cloth, leather was also used for the sleeveless 'buff' jerkin worn by many occupations. Originally worn by soldiers under their armour, this garment had first been made of buffalo hide, although the term now applied to various other leathers as well as to the colour. The leather was often oiled to increase its waterproof qualities and to make it pliable.

Some countrymen used aprons but shirt and breeches (*Plate 8, fig. 39*) on their own were usual in hot weather; in England men seldom worked in breeches alone.

Shepherds, and others who had to spend most of their time out of doors, kept warm and dry in various ways. Tabards, or tunics, of sheepskin were used by some Spanish shepherds; sleeveless, with the fleecy side out, they were longer at the back than the front and provided portable and damp-proof cushions when needed. In other parts of Europe similar warmth and protection was supplied by long unbelted coats and by 'over-all' garments or 'smocks'.

Leather shoes with wooden soles were in use, and in the Netherlands the wholly wooden shoe, clog or sabot, was worn by agricultural workers. (*Plate 7, fig. 32.*) These also cropped up in other parts of Europe when the ground was damp or muddy. In England at this time a swineherd, who also wore leather breeches, is recorded as having hob-nailed boots. Stockings without toes or heels were sometimes worn with the clogs, and poor people often put straw in them to keep their feet warm.

Heels appeared on shoes from about 1600 and were used by those working in towns, although flat soles were still to be seen. In southern Europe the strapped sandal was general. To protect the better type of shoes and to keep the wearer well clear of the mud, wooden soles on metal stands were strapped over the foot. (*Plate 7, fig. 35.*) However, these were not used when a great deal of walking had to be done.

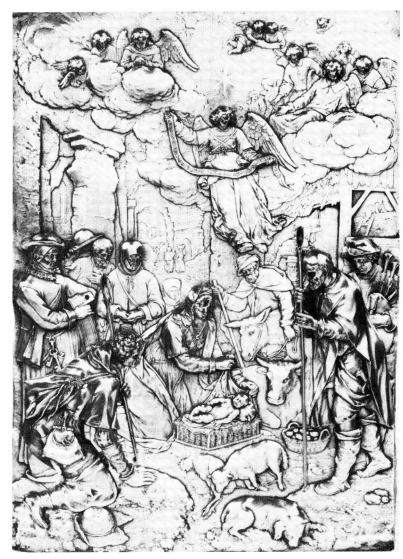

A Dutch silver plaque representing the visit of the shepherds to the infant Jesus. Note the scrip, or purse, worn by the shepherd on the left. (Paul van Vianen, 1607)

Gloves were now less common and were only used for special types of work, such as hedging and reaping.

Buttons of bone, metal and fabric were used for fastening but the poorer sections of the community still had to make do with pins, or even with long thorns.

Feudalism was at an end and peasants were beginning to own and work their small plots of land, although in certain parts of Europe they were still tied to a particular estate. But it meant that women now spent more of their time in the fields than they had previously done and, as a result, their skirts grew shorter. Almost without exception they wore aprons.

In the towns tradesmen's short aprons might be grey or white (*Plate 7, fig. 34, Plate 8, fig. 36*), although English weavers favoured green.

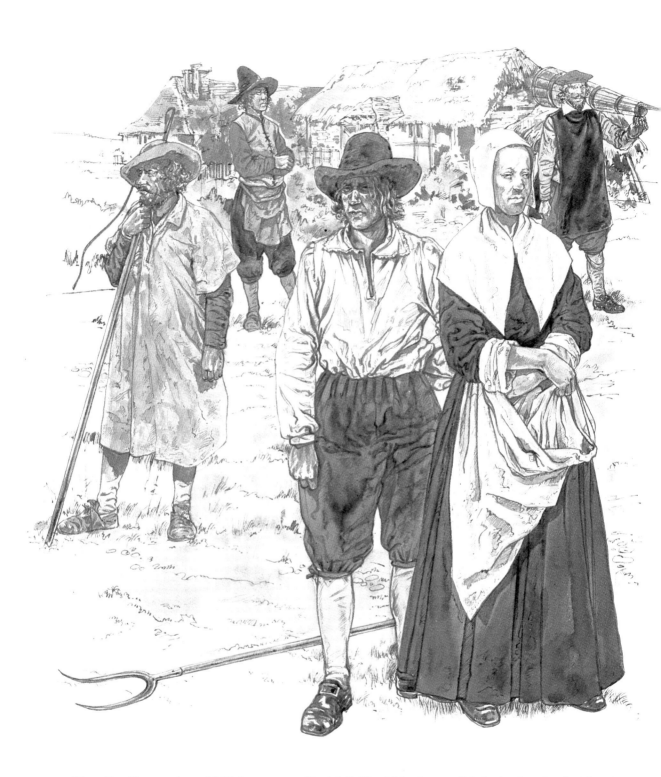

Plate 8 Chapter 4—mid 17th century (*Back left*) *Fig. 36* Innkeeper (Netherlands), (*Back right*) *Fig. 37* Water carrier (England), (*Front left*) *Fig. 38* Carter (England), (*Centre front*) *Fig. 39* Rural worker, haymaking (England), (*Front right*) *Fig. 40* Maid-servant (England).

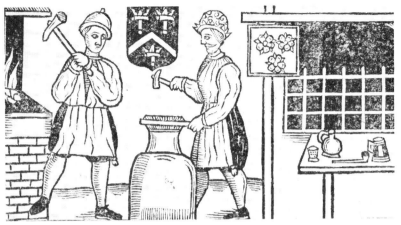

A woodcut of
blacksmiths at work.
(Manuscript 1660-1680)

Masons, blacksmiths and sometimes carpenters chose the greater protection of leather, as did miners in Germany who continued to use the back aprons of the previous century. These were combined with a sleeveless leather tunic and a hood. (*Plate 9, fig. 45.*)

As aprons were specifically a working garment for men they were discarded by them outside working hours. The Butchers' Company in London (who were so strict in their regulations that they even paid for apprentices' hair to be cut to an appropriate length) actually forbade members to wear aprons when not actually in their shops. Many butchers were now wearing oversleeves as well and these too were discarded when not in use. A number of tradesmen, including butchers, continued to wear close-fitting woollen caps.

Due to the increased interest in gardens (a fashionable addition to great houses now fortfications were no longer necessary) and to the introduction of new plants brought back by explorers, gardeners were now of considerable importance. Some even had their portraits painted dressed in the height of fashion. However, their working clothes were likely to be the usual breeches worn with a shirt and the sleeved, or sleeveless, jerkin. In the Netherlands this was another occupation which made use of wooden shoes.

A linen or canvas 'coat' that came into use during the seventeenth century was the forerunner of the smock. This, while it somewhat resembled the old tunic, differed from it because it was put on over other clothes to protect them and was, consequently, much more voluminous than either tunic or shirt. Coming well below the knee, it was soon adopted by men like shepherds and carters whose work kept them out in all weathers, and whose clothes were likely to be spoiled by mud or by the loads they carried. With a wide-brimmed hat and a long whip this smock now became the recognized dress of waggoners and carters, and was used for a very long time. (*Plate 8, fig. 38.*)

Although the number of independent workmen had greatly increased in towns and cities, wealthy folk still had large retinues of

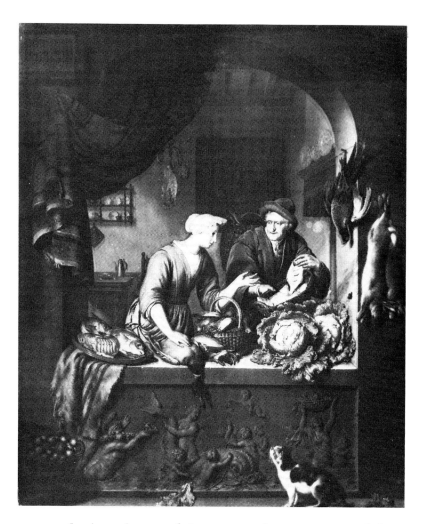

A poulterer's shop
painted by Mieris.
(1662-1747)

servants. In the early part of the seventeenth century many of them
were still dressed in livery, often blue like the clothes of other servitors.
Though virtually a uniform, livery had at least some advantages over
ordinary working dress; it was provided by an employer and was often
of better material than would otherwise have been available. Silk, for
instance, a fabric normally forbidden to working people, could be worn
by servants on the instruction of their master. However, even this was
insufficient to keep ambitious men in a standardized form of dress and
by the end of the century livery was only worn by those engaged on the
more menial tasks.

In the absence of livery, a badge enabled a servant to be recognized
when away from his employer's house—metal discs were attached to
sleeves of retainers such as watermen who otherwise might have found
it difficult to refuse to serve strangers. Such insignia was unnecessary
for indoor servants though some, in particular footmen, were to retain
livery long after others had abandoned it. This was possibly because

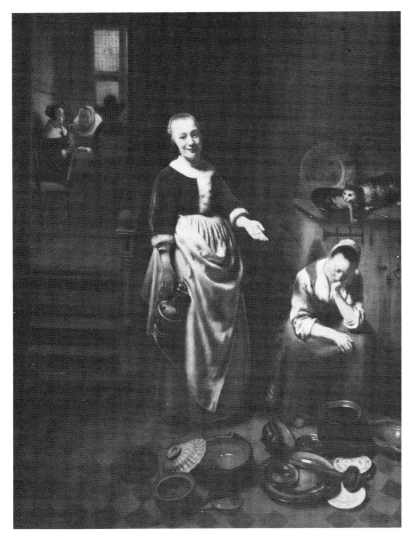

Two servants painted by
Nicolas Maes (1632-93)

their activities became increasingly ornamental rather than practical.
As a rule footmen's livery was close to fashionable dress and in 1666 the
king of France showed his scorn of the king of England by dressing his
footmen in the new fashion, petticoat breeches, that had just been
adopted by his brother monarch.

More women were now employed in private households but they
were never required to wear any kind of uniform. As a result, the same
criticism was made as was levelled at men servants when livery lost its
popularity; guests found it hard to tell them from members of the
family as their clothes were often equally fashionable. The only differences between those of many of them seems to have been that they wore
less costly fabric and used no fur trimmings. However, they did often
have long aprons and, in common with other working women, frequently a large unstarched kerchief or collar pinned at the neck. Like

country women, maid-servants looped up their overskirts while working so that the harder-wearing underskirt suffered any damage that might occur. A plain white head-dress was usually worn and the sleeves of the chemise were rolled back over the bodice sleeves. (*Plate 8, fig. 40*.) In hot climates like the Cape of Good Hope they wore sleeveless bodices (*Plate 7, fig. 33*) in place of the warmer sleeved versions more popular in northern Europe.

Both men and women now worked as cooks and wore long white bibless aprons over ordinary working dress, adding oversleeves to protect them from hot utensils and from the heat of the fire.

Street traders also made use of the long apron when selling food, although, on the whole, the clothes of these people, of whom there were many, were a collection of whatever garments could be gathered together for warmth. The picturesque appearance of the street trader has often been portrayed, but the clothes of many of the city 'cries' were simply derived from the rural dress of the area from which the individual had come. Some, as has been said, wore aprons and in London most of the men had long-sleeved, buttoned jackets or coats, with breeches and hose and large black felt hats.(*Plate 9, figs 41 & 42*.) Around their necks they often wore the knotted handkerchief that was becoming popular with other working men in town and country. (*Plate 9, figs 41 & 42*.) Most traders of this period are recognizable only from the wares with which they are festooned and which hung from belts or carried on their backs. Hat sellers, appropriately, carried many of their hats on their heads. One or two have specifically protective garments. A London coal trader suspended a length of cloth from his shoulders under his bag of coal, while a water-seller wore a very practical black leather tabard to protect him from splashes. (*Plate 8, fig. 37*.)

In London the name costermonger was given to traders who sold large apples called 'costards' and the term eventually came to apply to those who brought fruit, vegetables and fish from the large markets to sell in the street. At this period their dress appears to have differed little from that of other traders, though the women had shorter skirts and hats with flat crowns upon which they balanced their baskets. (*Plate 9, fig. 43*.) Some women traders in Paris were similarly attired.

Many goods were sold by these vendors and the confusion and noise must have been greatly increased as more coaches came into use and the streets grew busier: there were traffic jams even in the seventeenth century. Outdoor work of all kinds required protective clothing but coachmen sitting at the mercy of the elements for hours at a time had greater need of it than many. To ordinary working dress they began to add either a long and voluminous cloak, or a long and heavy coat, a wide hat, and strong, heavy boots, with large tops capable of being drawn right over the knee. Like the carter, the coachman carried a long whip as the symbol of his trade.

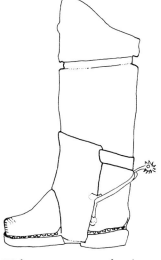

17th-century post-boy's boot.

Those who did not actually sell goods often advertised their services by the use of pictures. A rat catcher announced himself by a flag which in addition to being adorned with pictures had some dead rats hanging from it. A gelder wore a ribbon round his chest bearing pictures of horse shoes.

The streets were seldom empty during the day, but during epidemics they were likely to be deserted, although at night there was plenty of activity as bodies were carried away for burial under cover of darkness. During the Great Plague in London, in 1665, this task was carried out by men wearing the long gown with hanging sleeves that was more usually associated with doctors and scholars. Those medical men who remained in the city during the infection, and many did not, made some attempt to avoid contamination by enveloping themselves in huge tent-like garments of leather reaching to the ground. Over this they wore big gauntletted gloves and hoods that completely covered their faces, leaving only holes for the eyes. The most remarkable part of the costume, however, was a beak at the front of the hood which was filled with herbs to act as disinfectants.

Some moralists blamed the Plague, and the Fire that followed, on the materialism of the age. Certainly towards the end of the century clothes became richer and more colourful again which was partly due to the prosperity brought about by continued colonial expansion.

In the colonies themselves, however, clothes were much simpler. There, working people wore looser and lighter variants of what they had been used to at home. The sleeveless bodice, the skirt and the chemise for women, and the shirt, jerkin and breeches for men. Indigenous workers who did manual tasks for the settlers usually had their own costumes replaced by these garments, though they were not required to wear shoes. Conversely, Europeans in North America soon found that Indian moccasins were convenient for working in.

If changes in occupational and working dress came slowly in Europe they were even slower overseas where, due to the length of time taken on voyages, fashion changes were far behind those of Europe. Sailors, who spent much of their lives on these voyages, while they might dress reasonably fashionable on shore, had now developed a style of their own for the sea. There they favoured the earlier wide trousers or wore petticoats of canvas or sailcloth, tarred to make them weather-proof, over baggy breeches, or slops. Hats of fur and close-fitting woollen caps were still used, woollen mittens also helping to keep out wet and cold. Shirts were of brown or blue linen and covered with sleeved jerkins for warmth. Regulation clothing had begun to be issued but it was not until the nineteenth century that uniforms for sailors and for other occupations really became established.

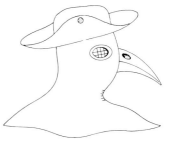

Protective mask worn by doctors attending Plague victims.

5 Industry versus agriculture

Dress differences in the mid-eighteenth century

A LOT OF THINGS ALTER in the course of a hundred years but so many new ideas, new attitudes and new methods came into being during the eighteenth century that it has often been called the Age of Enlightenment.

When the century began, Western Europe was almost completely agricultural, by the time it ended, commercial life and industry had begun to take the shape we know today.

At the very root of the changes was a desire for freedom of thought and action that sprang from a general disillusionment with the rule of prince and noble, disillusion that was eventually to lead to the American War of Independence and the French Revolution. Many developments in industry, and commerce too, came from dissatisfaction with the established order.

Of the inventions thought up by enlightened minds, many, like improved looms and spinning machines, were to do with the production of cloth for clothing. It is not to be wondered that the manufactories of the previous centuries continued to grow, like the towns that were spreading around them.

Although the majority of working people in Europe were still engaged in agriculture, the number of factory workers of all kinds increased. A vast number, particularly in England, also worked as servants. The eighteenth century saw, too, the emergence of a new type of worker, the public servant; for it was from now on that the postal and transport services really grew.

Basic working dress for men was still a shirt, with a jacket or jerkin, waistcoat, breeches and stockings, with hats or caps worn indoors and out. Though there was not a lot of difference in the basic garments of those at work in the town and those in the country, townsmen did manage to follow fashion more closely. Not quite the same thing happened with women's clothes, however, for by the middle of the eighteenth century there were beginning to be differences in rural costume from region to region, while urban dress developed certain characteristics of its own. On the whole, the differences came about through variations of the same garments.

The upper garment particularly popular with working women took two forms, one a short fitted jacket, and the other a gown which might be either short and loose, or long and more fitting. The gown, apparently, was the more popular in eighteenth-century England. So

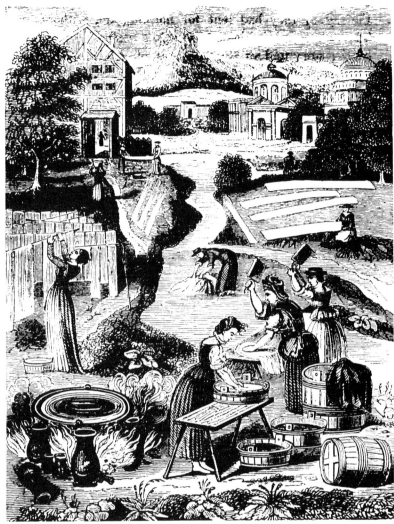

English laundresses at work with bare feet and bunched-up skirts. (English late 18th-century engraving)

convenient were these garments to work in when cool weather made them necessary that they continued in use into the nineteenth century. The short, loose gown had a wrap-over front and was often kept in place by an apron.

The clothes of both rural and urban working men in North America resembled those of their counterparts in Europe, though they were often of better fabric as they tended to be better off and better able to follow fashion. The clothes of the American womenfolk, however, particularly in rural areas, often seem to have been those of the region in Europe from which they had come.

The smock—a garment that is usually associated with farm labourers—began to justify this association towards the end of the century. A descendant of the tunic, the garment had already been in use in some parts of Europe but not specifically by country folk, being popular mainly with carters and shepherds. Although eventually widely used by male farm labourers in southern England, it was not confined to that region as different forms of it appear in Wales, in continental Europe, in America and even in the Cape of Good Hope.

Although one or two instances exist of the smock having been worn by women, it was really a masculine garment and remained such. Something like a modern-day overall, the labourer's smock had full-length sleeves and came to below the knees. It took various forms but always remained essentially practical. Made from a width of fabric, the fullness was gathered back and front, a large collar often giving extra protection to the shoulders from both weather and the friction of implements and loads. Chiefly of homespun linen that was very hard-wearing, the smocks varied considerably in both colour and style. Some were the same back and front, being slipped over the head with the cleaner side forward; others had a neck opening with a button, while yet a third type was open down the front with button fastenings. Often treated with oil to keep out the wet, they were known by a number of names: frock, slop-frock, smock-frock or smock. (*Plate 12, fig. 60.*)

Under his smock the countryman wore the usual working man's shirt, waistcoat and breeches, the latter sometimes of leather. The breeches' ties were often left open to make movement easier; woollen stockings reached to the knee.

As has been mentioned, the smock was also worn in the colonies, although in very hot weather it was usually discarded. In North America labourers and plantation workers wore only short trousers that came to just below the knee and were known as skilts.

Coats or jackets were sometimes replaced with a sleeved waistcoat, without a skirt if the flaps below the waist were likely to be inconvenient. Large overcoats, or surtouts, were worn in cold weather by prosperous country folk. A German farmer, towards the end of the century, was depicted with a coat of this kind, a wide-brimmed hat cocked on one side, breeches, stockings and buckled shoes.

The dress of French rural workers appears to have been very similar to that of their English counterparts, although womens' clothes tended to have more regional differences.

One notable change in the dress of farm labourers from earlier periods was that they appear to have abandoned the apron completely. This is perhaps accounted for by the increased popularity of an even more effective means of protecting the clothes and person—the smock.

Large, floppy, felt hats continued to be used to shield the head from rain and sun and to provide a certain amount of protection for neck and shoulders.

Gaiters of both leather and cloth were worn throughout Europe by all who needed extra protection and footless hose, sometimes quite loose and baggy, were also still in use.

Shoes had not changed a great deal. Country folk wore them laced or

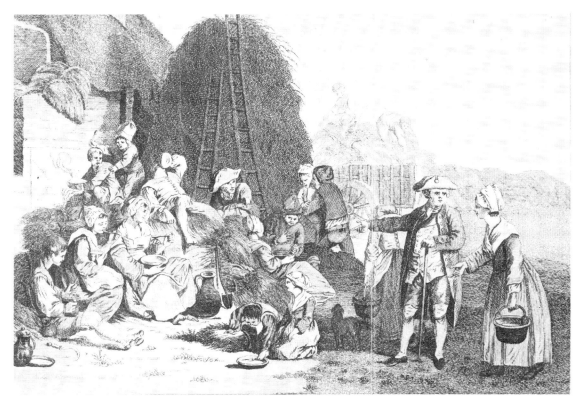

tied, the soles often reinforced with iron nails. Soles and heels might be of wood and the wooden clog was still widespread in France, Germany and the Netherlands. Although known in England, its use was not extensive as men favoured a short, laced boot known as a 'high-low' while women wore pattens, platforms of wood or metal, over their normal footwear. Foreign travellers observed that as a general rule country people in England were better shod than those on the European continent.

An eighteenth-century farmer with his reapers. (French engraving)

Town occupations were on the increase and although clothes had to be functional they were fairly close to fashionable wear but simplified, and of coarser and more hard-wearing materials. Coats were usually longer than those of country people, with more fabric and more elaborate cuffs. Tradesmen were prosperous and their grandeur in London can be judged by the fact that they could be distinguished by their white silk stockings. In general they wore jackets and waistcoats, breeches, stockings, a neckcloth and, almost invariably, an apron. Butchers who also wore oversleeves had already begun to use the blue ones that were to become their symbol; when actually in their shops they usually discarded their jackets and worked in sleeveless waistcoat, putting a close-fitting cap on their head in place of a hat. Most aprons were waist height but some were longer and had a bib fixed to a waistcoat button. (*Plate 11, figs 52 & 54.*) (*Plate 12, fig. 58.*)

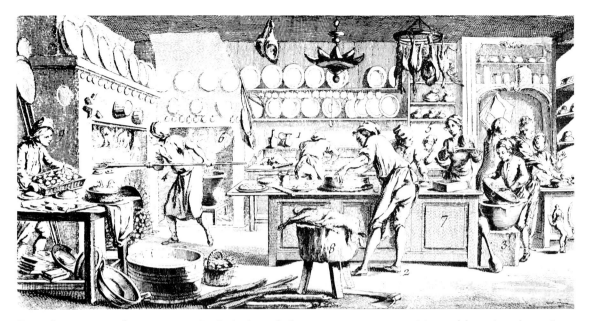

French pastry cooks
wearing caps and bibless
aprons. (Denis Diderot
*Encyclopedia of Trades
and Industry*, 1771)

In their shops bakers wore aprons over shirt and breeches, but when at their ovens sometimes only a loincloth. In North America towards the end of the century they are recorded as having 'plaited' aprons tied with a blue sash, while gunsmiths had green baize, and coopers and cordwainers white leather.

Town labourers worked in shirt and breeches with a waistcoat. (*Plate 12, fig. 57.*)

A lot of trading continued to be done in the streets and here, as in rural occupations, protection from the elements was the chief consideration and often entailed putting on several coats, or several pairs of stockings one over the other. A long coat and breeches were worn by men, while a jacket and several skirts tucked up out of the way were worn by women. Both usually wore wide-brimmed hats.

Many paintings of city 'cryes' in London, Paris and New York were done at this time but, as previously, although they gave some idea of the garments, most are probably more romantic than realistic. It is likely that most of their clothes were not only dirty but decrepit.

Milk and water sellers were a necessary part of the life of every city but, surprisingly enough, in spite of the leather aprons of some of their predecessors, in the eighteenth century they seldom seem to have bothered with protective clothing. For carrying their buckets watermen used hoops or frames hanging from straps over their shoulders and, as these kept the buckets well away from the body, they probably found further protection unnecessary. In America they wore leather breeches which certainly would have been more waterproof than cloth ones. Milkmaids carried their pails hanging from yokes that fitted across the shoulders, when not in use these were worn diagonally across the body. Like most other working women, milkmaids had white bibless aprons and white caps. Over the caps some wore black taffeta hats, though in London the milkmaids were noted for their straw hats decorated with flowers. (*Plate 10, fig. 47.*)

Working women still wore hooded cloaks out-of-doors and in England red ones were popular. Caps or kerchiefs were worn as well, and sometimes a hat. Almost all women street traders wore aprons either of blue, or white, and sometimes both together.

If street traders dressed mainly for warmth, those who sold in shops in the eighteenth century were more concerned with a fashionable appearance and, being better off, were more able to afford it. In fact, many employers even insisted that their assistants powdered and curled their hair in the latest styles.

The bright colours of servants' liveries must have added considerably to the gaiety of the streets for they might range from yellow, faced with black, to pale blue. These would be toned down, however, if they were in mourning for some member of their employer's family.

Footmen's liveries of collarless knee-length coats and plush breeches, with silk stockings and buckled shoes, began by following the fashion of the day. But as they remained in use when fashion changed they became fossilized, continuing to be used in a similar form right up to the present day. An addition to the footman's dress was the shoulder knot which was also to continue for a long time. This bunch of ribbon, or braid, had been worn by men of fashion as an ornament in the late sixteen hundreds and reappeared now on the left shoulder of footmen.

Like footmen, coachmen, postillions and grooms wore livery, although their breeches were frequently of leather and they had heavy boots. In the bad weather, to which they were so often subjected, coachmen used large overcoats with several capes to protect their shoulders. When their duties included rubbing down the horses they were likely to be issued with linen 'frocks' to protect their other garments. Grooms often had sleeved waistcoats with stripes and peaked caps. (*Plate 12, fig. 59.*)

When the Hanoverian kings came to the throne of England a black cockade was worn on the hat by officers in the army and navy. This was subsequently adopted, first by their livery servants, and then by those of many aristocratic families.

The drivers of stage coaches also wore caped coats, heavy boots and cocked hats. In North America in very cold weather these were exchanged for fur coats and fur hats.

A man-servant whose somewhat fantastic costume was more functional than it at first appears was the running footman. So-called because not only did he run ahead of a coach to give advance warning of his master's approach but he also literally ran errands. Though he belonged chiefly to the eighteenth century his clothes were more like those of the seventeenth century with petticoat breeches or a fringed skirt, the looseness of these garments making them ideal for running. The heavy fringes were necessary, however, because the running foot-man seldom encumbered himself with underwear. His clothes were light in fabric and also in colour to enable him to be seen more easily in the dark. Soft heel-less shoes added to his speed and a long staff helped him over ditches and streams. The staff usually had a round silver top that could be unscrewed to provide refreshment in the form of a hard-boiled egg or a small quantity of white wine. (*Plate 10, fig. 50.*)

Although otherwise dressed in ordinary coat and breeches worn with a peaked cap, foot messengers in France also wore heel-less shoes and carried long staffs. (*Plate 11, fig. 55.*)

A less functional and even more fanciful garb was that worn by the many black pages. These young boys, mostly slaves, were always dressed in a very elaborate way, their coats and breeches being of rich fabrics and gaudy colours with a great deal of trimming, and with a feathered turban. Any pride their elegant clothes may have given them must, however, have been dispelled by the silver collar, engraved with their master's name, that they wore round their necks. (*Plate 10, fig. 48.*) Pages dressed like this were to be seen in many parts of Europe, while in the Cape Colony one such youngster, in coat and breeches with stockings and heeled shoes, also wore a fashionably curled and powdered wig.

Servants' clothes generally tended to be better than anything they would have been able to afford in any other occupation, although this was not the case with inn servants. There were many more of these now as improved transport had increased the number of travellers but they were, as a rule, very poorly clad, except that most did wear aprons. In North America they, and their masters, who were often retired sol-diers, were able to afford rather better clothing.

Aprons were still the only occupational garments worn by women servants. Most of these just came to the waist (*Plate 10, fig. 49*) until the middle of the century when they began to have bibs. (*Plate 11, fig. 53.*) Bibless aprons were also worn with ordinary working dress by nursemaids in both England and France. Nursing was not yet the dignified profession it was to become and there was no specific form of clothing. Nurses dressed like other working women with, very occasionally, a badge.

More people were now engaged in industry and, although most wore basic working clothes, there were some rare instances of protective industrial clothing, some of which was surprisingly efficient.

The smock has already been described as a protective garment for agricultural workers and carters, but it was also, in a somewhat shorter and fuller version, the usual wear of glass workers in France. It protected the wearer from the heat of the furnaces while at the same

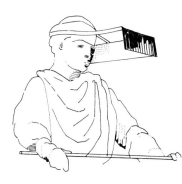

Eye shield worn in the 18th-century.

time enabling him to dispense with most of his other clothes, which he would have found much too hot. For extra protection these men sometimes added a rectangle of cloth tied round the neck and hanging down the front of the body. Where the eyes were likely to be at risk eye shields were used. Close-fitting caps were worn with these shields although many French industrial workers of the time favoured the large, wide-brimmed, felt hat; sometimes it was kept in place with a kerchief. Workers handling sheet glass wore enveloping leather overalls that covered both back and front of the body and stretched from neck to calf. (*Plate 12, fig. 56.*) In England, workers handling lead in the Wedgwood potteries also wore protective leather aprons.

Leather, of course, had been in use since ancient times to ward off sparks and heat and prevent clothing catching fire; aprons of blacksmiths, farriers and foundry workers were still being made in a similar manner to that in which the whole skin had been used. The farriers, like the slaughtermen, often used a sheepskin apron as well and wore wooden shoes. Many workers hung tools from their waists and French farriers are depicted with elaborate, pouched belts for the purpose.

Cloth aprons, sometimes with the bib fastened to a waistcoat button, were the sole concession to occupational dress by those who, like barbers, assisted the fashionable to remain in fashion. Otherwise they dressed in the latest style, avoiding very wide cuffs if they were likely to interfere with their work, but powdering their hair or wearing wigs as fashion dictated. (*Plate 12, fig. 58.*)

Public servants were on the increase and some were now wearing uniform. In the UK, red had long been the royal colour and was the obvious choice for the coats and heavy cloaks of the men employed by the Crown in the early years of the postal service. Firemen also were supplied with liveries or uniforms that varied according to the insurance company by whom they were employed. The uniforms usually followed the style of everyday dress. Watchmen, on the other hand, had no official costume but wore long and heavy belted greatcoats, with wide collars, and broad-brimmed hats, to keep them warm as they trudged about the dark streets with their lanterns and staffs.

Although they took considerable pride in their appearance when ashore, sailors still ignored fashionable styles when at sea; they continued to wear wide trousers and double-breasted jackets with handkerchiefs loosely knotted around their necks. (*Plate 10, fig. 46.*) At sea they wore a variety of hats, including ones of fur, but close-fitting knitted red caps were particularly popular.

About the middle of the century, British naval officers began to wear blue coats, while a certain amount of uniformity also became apparent among ships' crews.

Fishermen also favoured trousers and woollen caps and had oiled leather boots reaching to the knee, or just above. In France some fisher-

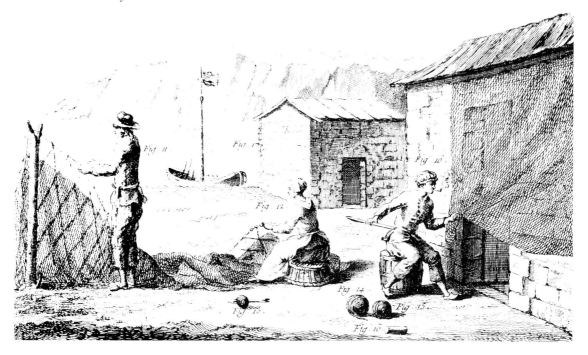

French fishermen and
fishwife. (Denis Diderot
*Encyclopedia of Trades
and Industry*, 1771)

men wore footless leggings and, occasionally, oval, wooden 'snowshoes'
to keep them from sinking in soft sand.

Although they did not actually go to sea, the clothes of fisherwomen
had a tendency to be different from those of other working women.
Their dress in Devonshire in the eighteenth century was described by a
contemporary as 'barbarous' chiefly because their skirts were, with
great practicality, looped up to form breeches. Some fisherwomen in
continental Europe adopted the same method to keep dry and move
about more easily than ankle-length skirts would generally allow. Most
went barefoot by the sea, although they wore shoes and frequently an
apron when selling fish.

Of all occupational dress, that of divers is certainly the most functional, for without it they would be unable to do their work. Diving
had been practised since ancient times and diving goggles are believed
to have been used in the second century. Over the years various kinds of
bells had been invented, but in the eighteenth century actual diving
suits were used with metal helmets, leather jackets and short leather
trousers.

Professional men in Europe and North America during the period
seem to have been sufficiently wealthy to dress in rich fabrics although
they chose sombre colours. By continuing to wear wigs long after they
had gone out of fashion they followed the tradition of appearing to
belong to an earlier and more dignified generation.

It is hard to say whether the dress of members of the legal profession,
which by the eighteenth century was already following a strictly

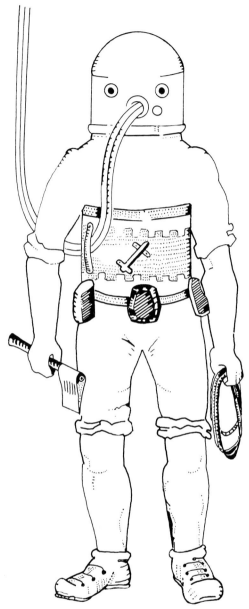

18th-century diving
apparatus.

hierarchial form, was uniform or occupational dress. Possibly it was
neither, because by this time it no longer served any function but was
purely traditional, as it has remained until the present day. Lawyers
already wore black robes in court at this period, while the scarlet gown
of the judge was another instance of the use of the royal colour for a
Crown official.

Physicians continued to dress in black, but they had adopted some
occupational garments for they wore close-fitting skull caps, aprons
and oversleeves for operations.

6 Occupations advertised

Colourful clothes 1789–1840

THE LATE EIGHTEENTH and early nineteenth centuries are rich in examples of colourful occupational costume for there have been few periods when, in a crowded street, the observant person could so easily tell the trade of those who passed by.

There were, fortunately, many of these observant people who used their talents to record the varied cavalcade. The fact that they wished to do so was partly due to a new awareness of the differences between the classes and between the elaborate clothes of the wealthy and the more practical garments of the working people. In Europe, North America and the colonies, at least in the cities and towns, the clothes of workers were very similar. Although regional differences were emerging these tended to be confined to rural areas and had little to do with occupation.

Industrialization continued faster than ever. New machines were being developed to produce more and more goods, and methods of transport improved to carry them from place to place. Much of the expansion was in the cloth industry and, after centuries of having little choice of fabric apart from what they made at home, poorer people were now benefiting as the range of cheap fabrics increased and were widely marketed. The first department stores opened, the first commercial travellers took to the road, and advertising began to appear in the new cheap press.

The fact that there was an increase of approximately 40% in the world population between 1800 and 1840 meant that not only was more labour available but also that there was a greater demand for the goods produced. In addition, the old self-sufficient village ways were dying out and cottage industries fast disappearing. On account of this, more women were now working on the land as farming became profitable for those who could afford to take advantage of new methods. Women were also working in the mines and in the mills, achieving an independence which may well have begun to arouse a desire for similar independence in the minds of their better educated sisters, for whom, up till now, the only respectable way of earning a living was as a governess.

Basic working dress for men continued to be shirt, waistcoat (with or without sleeves) and breeches. Trousers were only gradually being adopted by working men in England though they had been worn in Scotland since the banning of the kilt in 1746 and were also, with a short jacket and wooden shoes, the dress of the French labourer.

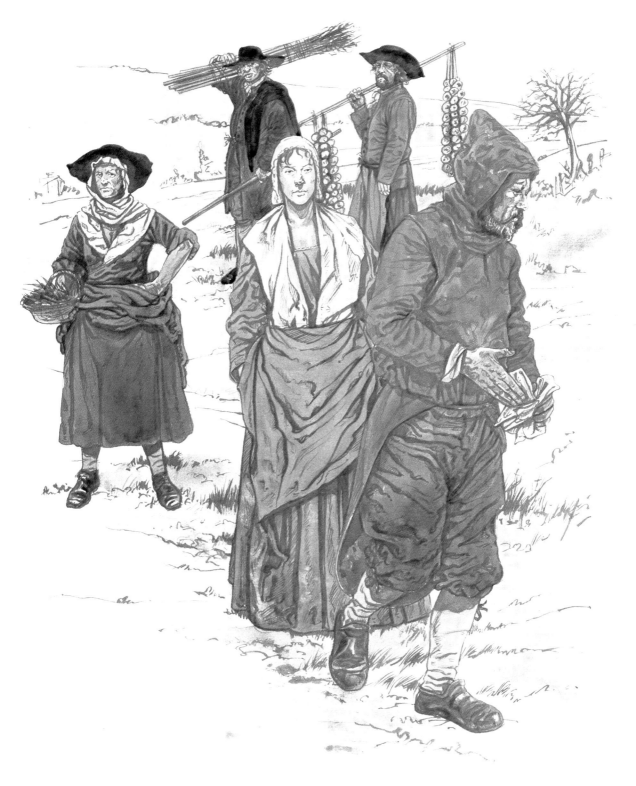

Plate 9 Chapter 4—late 17th century (*Back left*) *Fig. 41* Sweep (England), (*Back right*) *Fig. 42* Street trader (England), (*Front left*) *Fig. 43* Street trader (England), (*Centre front*) *Fig. 44* Maid-servant (England), (*Front right*) *Fig. 45* Miner (Germany).

Shirts, which were usually without a fastening, had a dropped shoulder line and were worn however hot the weather. Only miners stripped to the waist. Previously of flannel or coarse linen, these shirts were now frequently of cotton. In France some workers wore a blue blouse, rather like the smock of agricultural labourers and carters in England.

As more work was now being done under cover, wide-brimmed hats were less common although a headcovering of some kind was always worn. In France, following the Revolution, it was the 'cap of liberty', a descendant of the Phyrigian cap placed on the heads of freed slaves in Roman times.

Women still wore a gown and an apron over petticoat or chemise. Around their necks was a shawl or neckerchief, and on their heads a white cap, with a bonnet or straw hat for outdoor wear. Women doing field work often discarded their gowns and wore only their chemise with their stays, or corset bodice, on top of it. As this was not really an undergarment, removing the gown was considered no more indecent than removing the waistcoat and working in shirtsleeves was for men.

As had been the case hundreds of years earlier, the shepherd's flock continued to 'afford him his whole raiment', though seldom as literally as it did some Spanish shepherds who wore not only sleeved tunics of sheepskin but sheepskin trousers as well. (*Plate 14, fig. 66.*) In other countries sheepskin waistcoats were worn with woollen jackets and breeches, or with leather breeches. Shepherds needed not only protection against the elements but often against parasites as well. In some central European countries they solved the problem by boiling their shirts and trousers in lard and by smearing themselves with the same commodity. Just as well, perhaps, that they spent much of their lives away from the rest of humanity!

In both Europe and North America, leggings or gaiters helped to keep out cold and damp, being made of various kinds of strong cloth, canvas, linen, wool and leather. They tied below the knee and also at the ankle, or buttoned or buckled down the outside of the leg. Shepherds and other farm workers also used twists of straw for the purpose, a practice still to be current a hundred years later. Leggings extending over the instep were known as spatter-dashes.

Shoes and boots of leather were worn but in France, parts of England and Wales wooden clogs or wooden-soled shoes continued. In Scotland, instead of being made to keep out the damp, some boots had small holes pierced in the soles to let water escape.

Various items that might be considered tools or garments were to be seen in the countryside at this time, including leg and knee pads, gloves and sowing sheets. The latter were now put on over the shoulder and wrapped round the arm to form a pouch for holding seed. (*Plate 16, fig. 80.*)

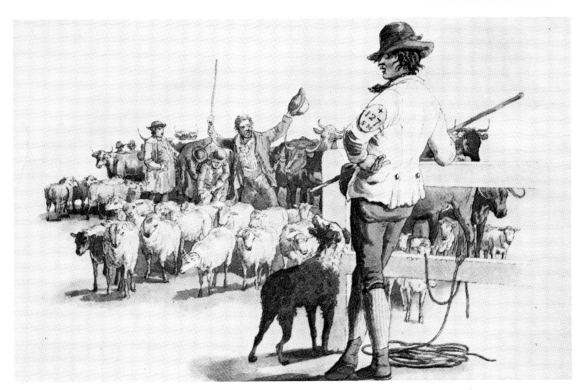

Clothes to protect workers from early machines were lacking and there must have been many accidents due to unsuitable garments. Factories and mines had large numbers of employees, and often very young children earned a living by doing simple tasks such as opening and shutting the doors in underground shafts, sometimes entirely naked or dressed only in a loincloth. Girls and women were also employed underground, many of them wearing trousers and nothing else apart from a leather belt holding the chains by which they dragged coal carts through the narrow passages. Men also worked naked, or in trousers alone, although some wore the basic working dress of shirt and breeches. In some places, however, white jackets and breeches were worn. (*Plate 14, fig. 67.*) This may have been because, needing frequent washing they encouraged hygiene, but it is possible that they made the workers more easily seen underground, reflecting as they did what little light came from candles and primitive lamps.

In most factories people wore their ordinary clothes, though women and children sometimes had pinafores (*Plate 16, fig. 76*) and male factory workers were among those who adopted the increasingly popular paper hat. (*Plate 16, fig. 77.*) Some factories employed large numbers of children who lived on the premises and were clothed and fed. One such factory in Scotland supplied its child workers with cotton garments in summer and woollen ones in winter.

Another vast army of unskilled labourers were the navvies, or inland

A drover wearing a numbered arm-band. In the background on the left there is a farmer in a smock. (W. H. Pyne, *Costume of Great Britain*, 1805)

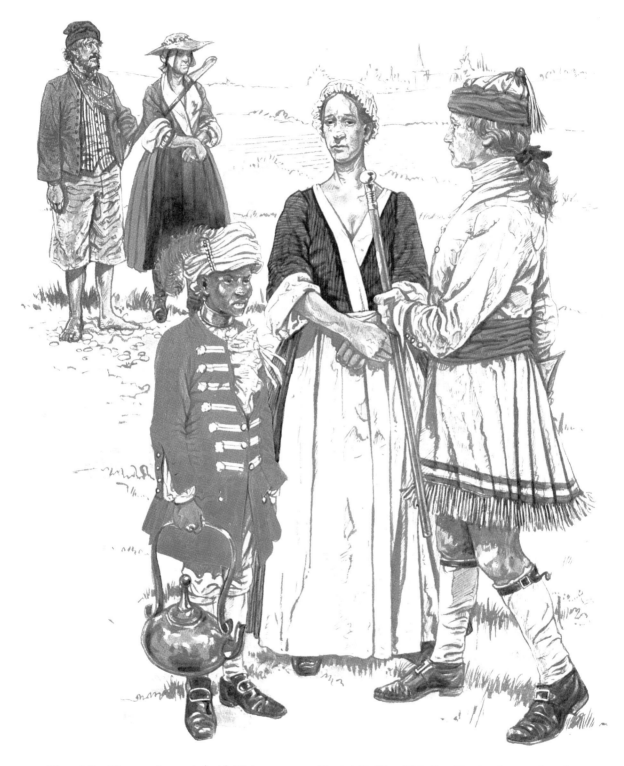

Plate 10 Chapter 5—early/mid 18th century *(Back left) Fig.* 46 Sailor (England), *(Back right) Fig.* 47 Milkmaid (England), *(Front left) Fig.* 48 Negro page (England), *(Centre front) Fig.* 49 Maid-servant (England), *(Front right) Fig.* 50 Running footman (England)

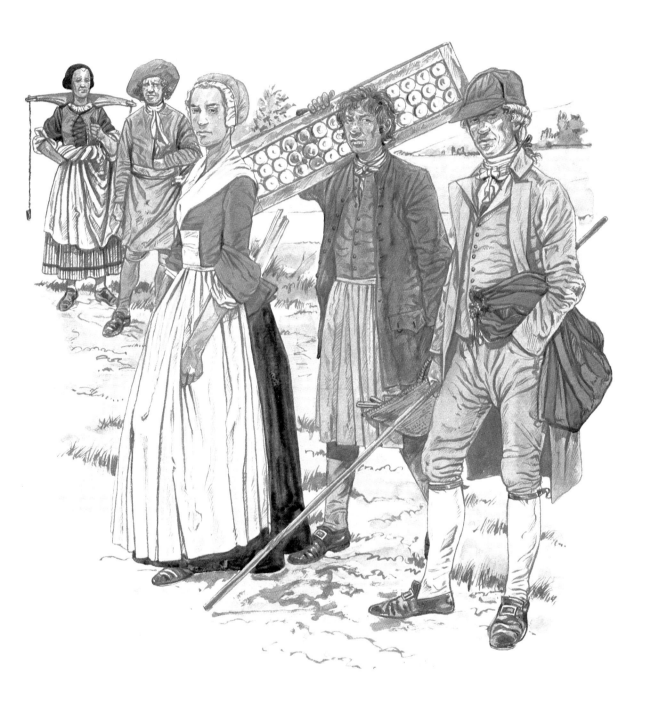

Plate 11 Chapter 5—mid 18th century (*Back left*) *Fig. 51* Milkmaid (Germany), (*Back right*) *Fig. 52* Tradesman (Netherlands), (*Front left*) *Fig. 53* Maid-servant, (*Centre front*) *Fig. 54* Glazier (Italy), (*Front right*) *Fig. 55* Messenger (France).

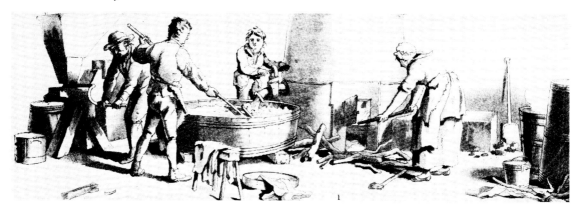

Cider-makers with hide aprons over their ordinary working dress. (W. H. Pyne, *Microcosm*, 1808)

navigators, so called because a great many were engaged in digging canals for the extension of the inland waterways. In spite of the fact that they were well paid according to the standards of the time, these men were among the roughest and most uncouth of the new industrial workers. Most wore trousers rather than breeches, woollen caps and shirts that, like others of the period, at least started off as white. (*Plate 14, fig. 70.*)

Red knitted caps, worn by navvies as well as the more popular striped ones, were known as brewers' caps because they were frequently worn by employees of the big English breweries. Draymen, who transported the beer, considered themselves further up the social ladder and favoured high-crowned hats. These men, like all drivers of horse-drawn vehicles, needed to be warmly dressed and usually wore square-cut cloth coats, reinforced with leather, warm waistcoats and leather aprons (*Plate 15, fig. 71*), though ordinary carters still retained their long smock.

Leather aprons were also worn, as they had always been, by black-smiths and farriers. (*Plate 15, fig. 74.*)

A raw hide apron was usually added to a leather one to provide the butcher's slaughterman with additional protection in his messy and often dangerous job. Leather leg shields, or pads, were added to save his legs from the hooves of the animals he had to dispatch. (*Plate 13, fig. 63.*)

Breeches still remained the choice of tradesmen who, like labourers, frequently discarded their coats and worked in shirt and waistcoat. Aprons, though now seldom used by labourers, were still indispensable to shopkeeper and tradesman and remained so until the arrival of the overall.

These aprons usually fell from the waist but where tools or materials were likely to touch the upper part of the body, as with carpenters and coopers, they might be attached to shirt or waistcoat button. Coopers were also one of the trades who made use of protective oversleeves. (*Plate 15, fig. 73.*)

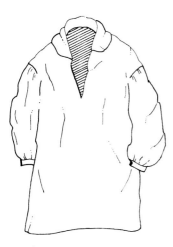

19th-century carter's smock.

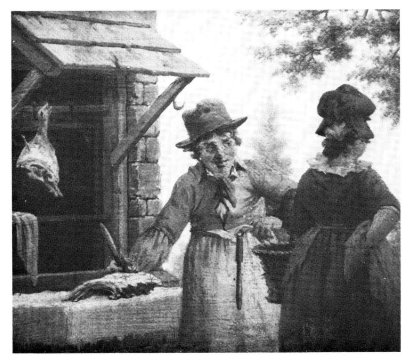

Butcher in white apron.
(Early 19th-century
painting by John Cranch)

Butchers, understandably enough, also wore oversleeves of washable fabric in either blue or white. In England from the end of the eighteenth century blue was also the usual choice for aprons, no doubt because blood stains, which so often remain after washing, are less noticeable on blue than on white.

Because of the open fronts of their shops most butchers wore either sleeved waistcoats, or blue cloth coats, and heavy top-boots, sometimes keeping their heads warm with brewers' caps or, when it became fashionable, with the ubiquitous top-hat.

In other shops, particularly those dealing in clothes or the accessories of dress, assistants were expected to be neatly and reasonably fashionably clad; women usually wore black aprons, often of satin.

Shops continued to increase in number but street traders still sold many of the staple foods. Among the men, some wore trousers and some breeches, but all clung to the floppy black hats of the previous period. Women's headgear was more varied, both hoods and hats were sometimes worn at the same time. (*Plate 13, fig. 61.*) Some London milkmaids in the 1820s wore black top-hats, the now less common corset bodice, and very short skirts. A more usual sight was probably the milkmaid in a short-sleeved gown with bunched up skirt that showed her chemise, and a flat straw hat over a mob-cap. (*Plate 13, fig. 64.*) Some milk sellers did the milking themselves and the cap, or a hood, which they wore under their hats served to protect the hair when their heads rested against the cow's flank.

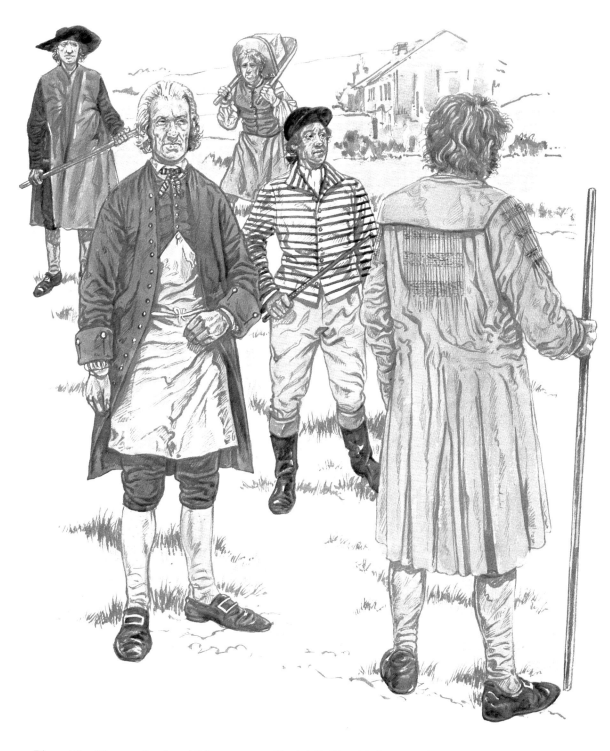

Plate 12   Chapter 5—late 18th century   (*Back left*) *Fig. 56* Glass worker (France), (*Back right*) *Fig. 57* Stonemason (France), (*Front left*) *Fig. 58* Barber (England), (*Centre front*) *Fig. 59* Groom (England), (*Front right*) *Fig. 60* Farm labourer (England).

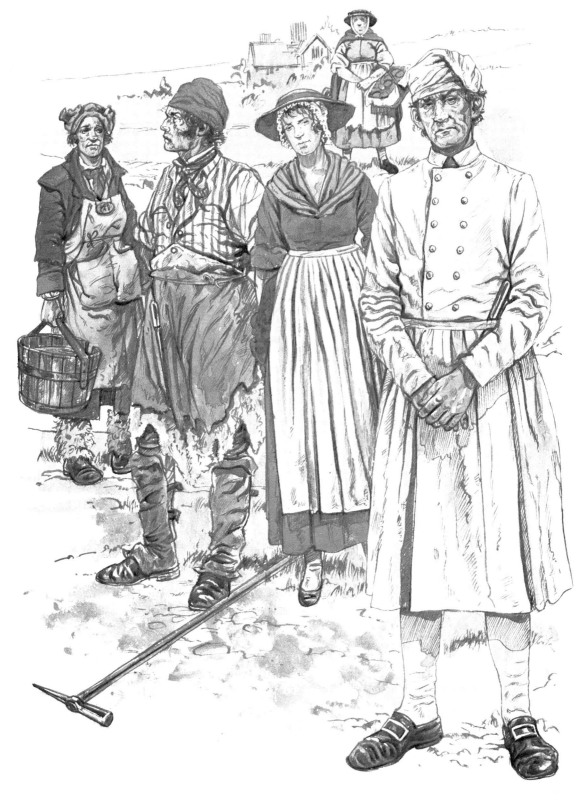

Plate 13 Chapter 6—early 19th century (*Back right*) *Fig. 61* Street trader (England), (*Back left*) *Fig. 62* Hackney coachstand waterman (England), (*Front left*) *Fig. 63* Slaughterman (England), (*Centre front*) *Fig. 64* Milkmaid (England), (*Front Right*) *Fig. 65* Cook (England).

Occasionally, the street vendors carried heavy loads which they supported in various ways. The women salt vendors (one is tempted to call them salt sellers) of Scotland wore headbands to take the weight on their foreheads. This meant they had to wear hoods instead of hats.

The cleanliness, or otherwise, of streets was a serious problem but professional sweepers did their best to make a way through the mud for pedestrians. Although they seldom had any distinctive dress, in France some wore trousers with protective panels on the front and sides of the leg, jackets with a deep collar to protect the shoulders, wooden clogs and wide hats covering the back of the neck.

Hats with deep brims at the back to protect head and shoulders were one of the trademarks of the London dustmen who also had light coloured jackets, spatter-dashes (short gaiters), and heavy boots. These men carried large wicker baskets to remove the refuse, and bells to announce their arrival. The fan-tailed hats, as they were called, were also sometimes worn by draymen instead of the tall hats already mentioned, and by coal carriers.

Another occupation distinguished by its headgear, though for very different reasons, were the barbers. They, no doubt as a form of advertisement, wore the very latest fashions while remaining faithful either to the now old-fashioned wig or to powdered hair.

Wigs and powdered hair were also to remain a part of servants' livery for some time to come and, along with the eighteenth-century breeches, they continued to be worn by many servants long after not only men of fashion but the whole working population kept their hair natural and wore trousers.

One type of servant who probably found the wig a satisfactory way of

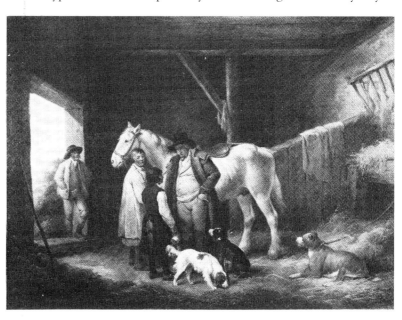

Dustman's hat worn in the 19th century.

An ostler and a pot boy dressed in different styles. (George Morland, 1763-1804)

keeping his head warm, for he often had to take off his hat, was the coachman. Sitting for hours on the box of a carriage he needed all the warmth he could get which, of course, was why he wore a heavy overcoat with a number of capes. Along with this garment he wore waistcoat, breeches and top-boots. (*Plate 16, fig. 78.*) Stagecoach drivers were similarly dressed, one writer describing them as wearing 'a multiplicity of coats' in which they were buried 'like cauliflowers'. Others were more dandified and contented themselves with two waistcoats. (*Plate 15, fig. 75.*)

Coaches had begun to carry the mails in England in 1784 and the first uniforms for employees of the Post Office were issued in 1793. Keeping the tradition of red for royal servants, the letter carriers and guards and drivers of mail coaches were provided with red coats that had blue lapels and cuffs; their waistcoats were blue and they were also supplied with yellow-trimmed beaver hats. (*Plate 15, fig. 72.*) Trousers they obtained for themselves. Suburban postmen had the colours in reverse—blue coats with red facings.

Some gentlemen of fashion drove their own light carriages in town: on the back of these elegant cabriolets balanced an equally elegant, though diminutive, ornament—the tiger. This small boy, whose main function seems to have been to hold the horse's head when his master dismounted, was probably so called because he wore the traditional yellow and black vertically striped waistcoat of a groom. Apart from his coat, which was often of some gorgeous hue, he wore the accoutrements of a groom, top-hat, top-boots and doeskin breeches. (*Plate 16, fig. 79.*)

In cities a variety of vehicles were beginning to ply for hire. Cab drivers and attendants at hackney stands usually wore caped coats and had neckerchiefs knotted round their throats. (*Plate 13, fig. 62.*) Chairmen (carriers of sedan chairs), where they still existed, also wore heavy coats and these sometimes had collars that could be buttoned so as to cover most of the face.

Horse omnibuses appeared in Paris in 1819 and in London some ten years later. To begin with the driver looked very much like the coachman of any private family, although the top-hat soon gave way to a more convenient peaked cap. Some enterprising proprietors equipped their coachmen with wooden bracelets on each arm to which long strings were attached. Passengers wishing to get down from the omnibus pulled the string on the side upon which they wished to dismount.

There was still no livery or uniform for women servants who wore simple gowns with large bibless aprons. However, the arrival of cheap cotton fabrics from North America resulted in the use of more prints. Scrubbing women and servants in small households still often wore the old-fashioned short gown with an ankle-length chemise (pinned up and worn with pattens for washing and scrubbing) and a neckerchief, with a

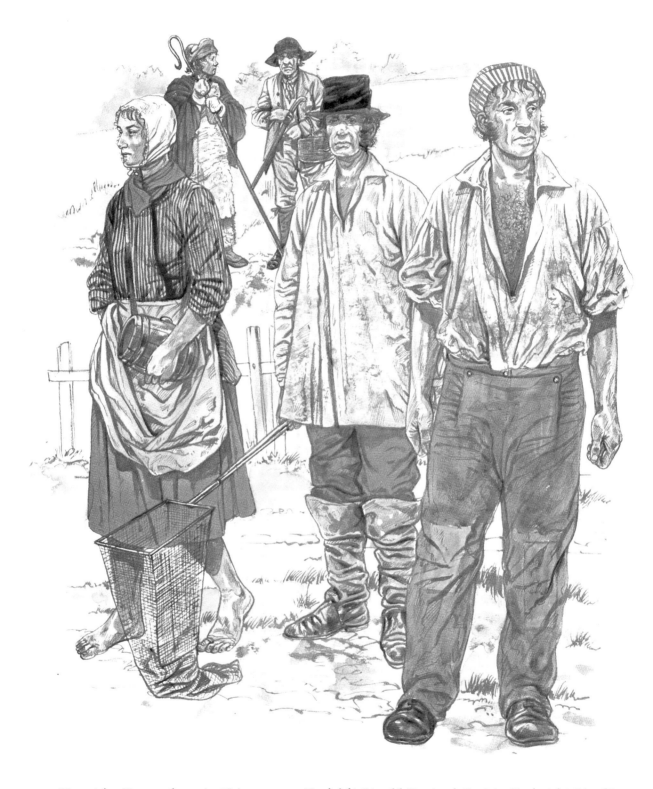

Plate 14   Chapter 6—early 19th century   (*Back left*) *Fig.* 66 Shepherd (Spain), (*Back right*) *Fig.* 67 Collier (England), (*Front left*) *Fig.* 68 Leech gatherer (England), (*Centre Front*) *Fig.* 69 Inshore fisherman (England), (*Front right*) *Fig. 70* Labourer (England).

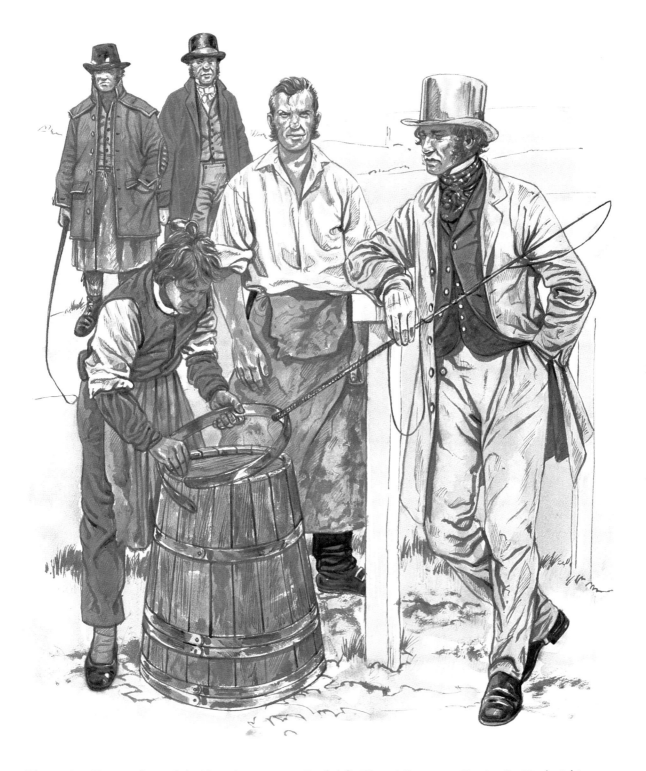

Plate 15 Chapter 6—early/mid 19th century (*Back left*) *Fig. 71* Drayman (England), (*Back right*) *Fig. 72* Postman (England), (*Front left*) *Fig. 73* Cooper (England), (*Centre front*) *Fig. 74* Blacksmith (America), (*Front right*) *Fig. 75* Coach driver (England).

mob-cap or a cap tied under the chin.

Nurserymaids and children's nurses wore cap and apron but no special form of clothing. On the European continent, however, as nurses were often drawn from rural areas, they frequently wore the dress of the region from which they came, or at any rate the head-dress that was peculiar to it.

Women cooks now predominated but in some large establishments the cooks were still men and they were beginning to wear white jackets with their aprons. (*Plate 13, fig. 65.*) By the 1820s the soft 'nightcap' was being replaced by a stiffened hat.

A form of apron, very unlike that of servants, was worn by seafaring men. This reached only to the knee and when treated with tar provided extra protection from the weather, and in the case of fishermen, from the catch. The sleeveless waistcoat, so widely worn by working men on land, did not provide a great deal of warmth for seamen, and as they did not wish to be encumbered with skirted coats these were no use either. Instead they adopted a form of waistcoat with sleeves that was known as a 'fearnothing' or 'dreadnought'. A similar garment was used by labourers who needed something more than the ordinary waistcoat. Wide breeches, or slops, were still worn by seamen although trousers were now commonplace. Oiled leather boots, which varied in length from mid-calf to thigh, were worn not only by sailors and sea fishermen in Europe and North America but also by those who lived by the produce of inland waterways. The fishermen of the low-lying fens of the east coast of England, living under such difficult conditions that they did not remove their clothes for weeks at a time, had boots that reached the thigh and they wore a smock rather than a jacket. (*Plate 14, fig. 69.*) Unlike the fenland fisherman, who might use a tall hat, seafarers wore close-fitting woollen caps.

At the start of the nineteenth century, as an alternative to water-proofing with tar, cloth as well as leather was being treated with oil and, as a result, 'oilskin' garments were beginning to be worn.

In many areas fisherwomen had a distinctive dress, the most notable feature of which was the shortness of the skirts—a necessity for women who spent much of their time in or near water. As a rule the gown was bunched up to show the petticoat beneath, and aprons were worn over these, although they too might be bunched up to the waist. Kerchiefs were usually worn tied underneath the chin, sometimes with soft-crowned bonnets or hats on top of them. Round their shoulders were shawls and, though they went barefoot by the sea, shoes and stockings were worn when selling fish.

A somewhat similar dress was that of women engaged upon the unpleasant task of collecting leeches. These creatures attached them-selves to the women's bare feet and legs and were then transferred to the small barrels which hung round their necks. (*Plate 14, fig. 68.*)

Due to the use which they made of the leech much of the work of doctors of the period involved the drawing of blood but, even during major operations, they seldom wore any kind of protective clothing at all. Black frock-coats were their usual wear whatever they were engaged upon, and the most they did before major surgery was to roll up their sleeves.

Members of the professions in general, like doctors and lawyers, were still inclined to see themselves as belonging to an earlier, more dignified age and continued to affect the dress of the previous generation. At the end of the eighteenth and the start of the nineteenth centuries they were, therefore, clinging with tenacity to the old-fashioned powdered wig, neatly tied at the back of the neck with a black ribbon.

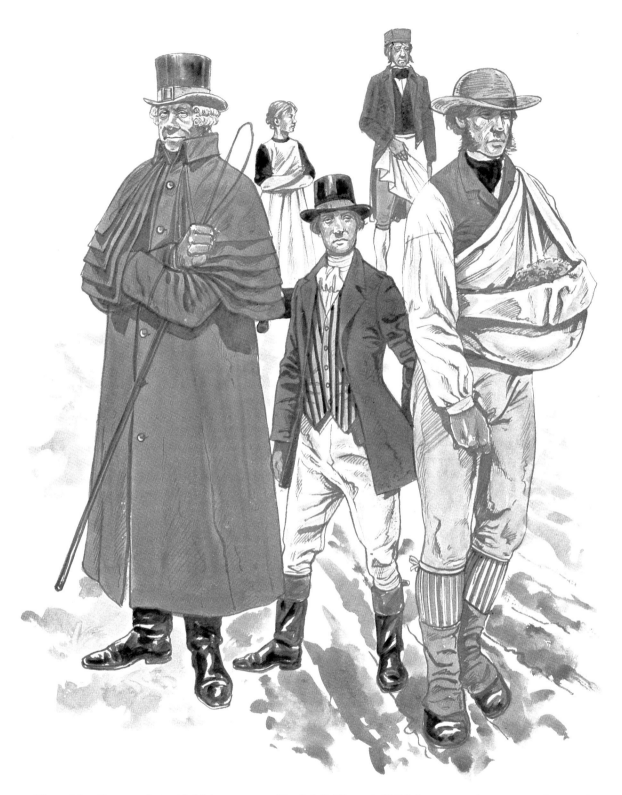

Plate 16 Chapter 6—mid 19th century (*Back left*) *Fig.* 76 Child factory worker (England), (*Back right*) *Fig.* 77 Factory worker (England), (*Front left*) *Fig.* 78 Coachman (England), (*Centre front*) *Fig.* 79 'Tiger'—young groom (England), (*Front right*) *Fig.* 80 Rural worker, sowing (England).

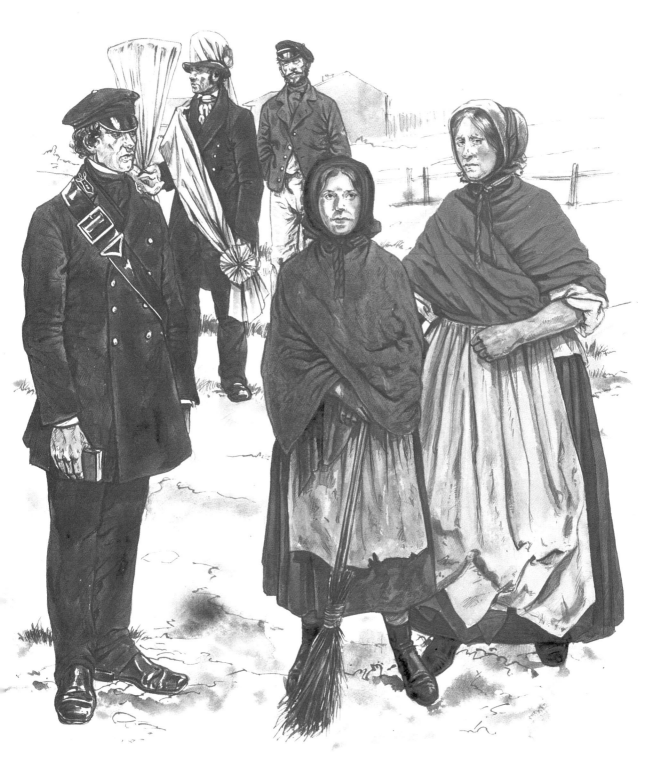

Plate 17   Chapter 7—mid/late 19th century   (*Back left*) *Fig. 81* Undertaker's mute (England), (*Back right*) *Fig. 82* Train driver (England), (*Front left*) *Fig. 83* Train guard (England), (*Centre front*) *Fig. 84* Child street sweeper (England), (*Front right*) *Fig. 85* Street trader (England).

7 Mills, mines and chimney-pot hats

1840–1890

ALTHOUGH OCCUPATIONAL COSTUME added colour to many periods it did so only in a purely nominal sense in the latter part of the nineteenth century. Dress in general was dark and dreary, and the smoke of railways and factories blotted out the bright colours of the previous decades leaving a gloomy grime encrusting all sections of society. And, as if to add to the illusion of industry, men, from dukes to zoo attendants and bootlace sellers, wore stovepipe and chimney-pot hats upon their heads.

There were, of course, many reasons why clothing had become so dark but one was certainly pollution of a kind that had never occurred before. Mud and soot were the inevitable consequences of industrial expansion—a price to be paid for wealth and progress—proving the old saying that where there was muck there was money.

Even those accumulating most of the wealth, the mine and mill owners, who could have afforded 'forty maids with forty mops' to keep them and their houses clean, did not indulge in bright colours. Black, brown and grey, enlivened by dark green and maroon, were relieved only by pastel prints and the white of shirts and aprons.

Although little of the wealth came the way of the ordinary working people there was an increase in the number and variety of jobs and, from the point of view of employers, it was just as well that the population increased at the same time.

The need for transport and services became greater as towns grew up around mines and factories, bringing offices, shops and many new white-collar occupations. Some of these suited women and, because a variety of work apart from domestic chores was becoming available to them, their status greatly improved towards the end of the century.

As a result women's working clothes became much more practical than ever before. In the past men's clothes had, since the adoption of the short tunic and hose, been well adapted for work but women's, because of long skirts, had not. During the nineteenth century this began to change as more women, becoming increasingly involved in work outside the home, found it convenient not only to shorten their skirts but in some cases to wear trousers. (The mere thought of these garments being worn by females was to horrify the great majority of people for nearly another century.)

With a few exceptions working men had now replaced breeches with trousers though, because it made movement easier and prevented them wearing out, they were often tied below the knee. With trousers went a shirt, now often coloured and sometimes of calico with linen collar and wrist bands, and a waistcoat either with or without sleeves. (*Plate 18, fig. 88 & Plate 20, fig. 96.*) Corduroy was even more widely used than before, though homespun still sometimes took its place, and a fabric called moleskin, a linen and cotton mix, was also popular. Real moleskins were occasionally used by gamekeepers for their waistcoats, although these were usually made of woollen cloth, velveteen or corduroy. Smocks remained popular for some occupations in the UK as did the workman's blue denim *blouse* in France. Caps were increasingly becoming the symbol of the working man, though top-hats were worn by some in the cities while in the country wide-brimmed hats of felt offered additional protection from the weather.

For most women the basic work dress was still a gown or a bodice, with a skirt and a chemise, or petticoat, beneath. Along with the indispensable white apron a plaid shawl was now added, with a bonnet, or sometimes a man's hat, and boots. (*Plate 18, fig. 87.*)

In spite of the many advances in agriculture, farming people still remained the most conservative in their dress, particularly in England where the eighteenth-century breeches and white shirt were still popu-

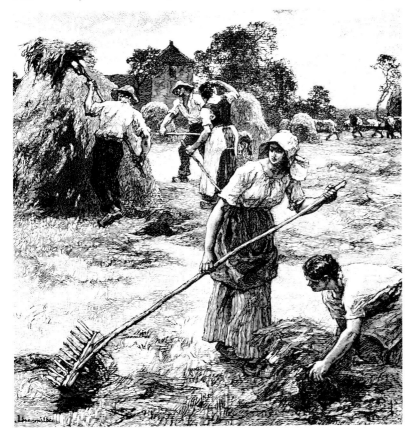

Harvesters. Woman in the centre wears a short-sleeved chemise and a sunbonnet. (*The Sunday Magazine*, 1889)

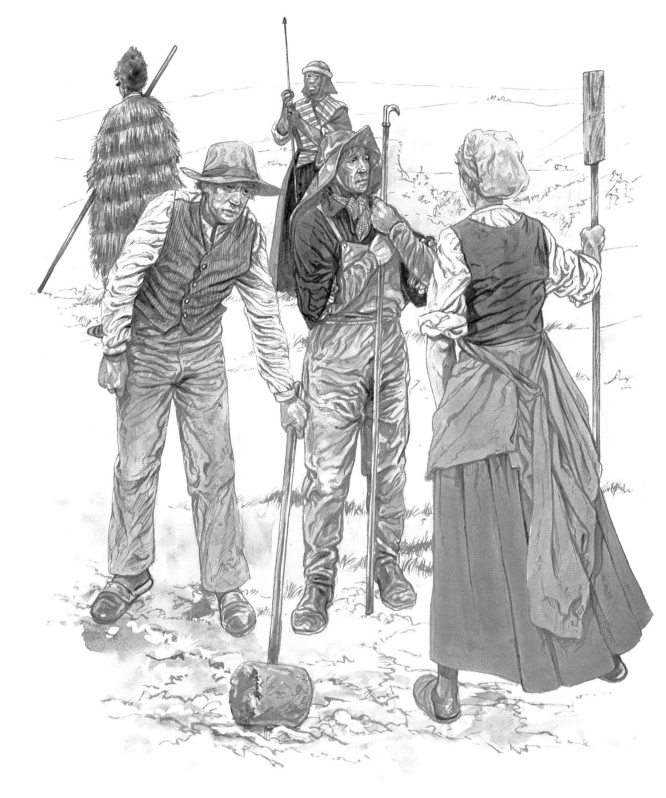

Plate 18   Chapter 7—mid/late 19th century   (*Back left*) *Fig. 86* Rural worker (Spain), (*Back right*) *Fig. 87* Negro servant (America), (*Front left*) *Fig. 88* Road worker (France), (*Centre front*) *Fig. 89* Fisherman (Netherlands), (*Front right*) *Fig. 90* Rural worker (France).

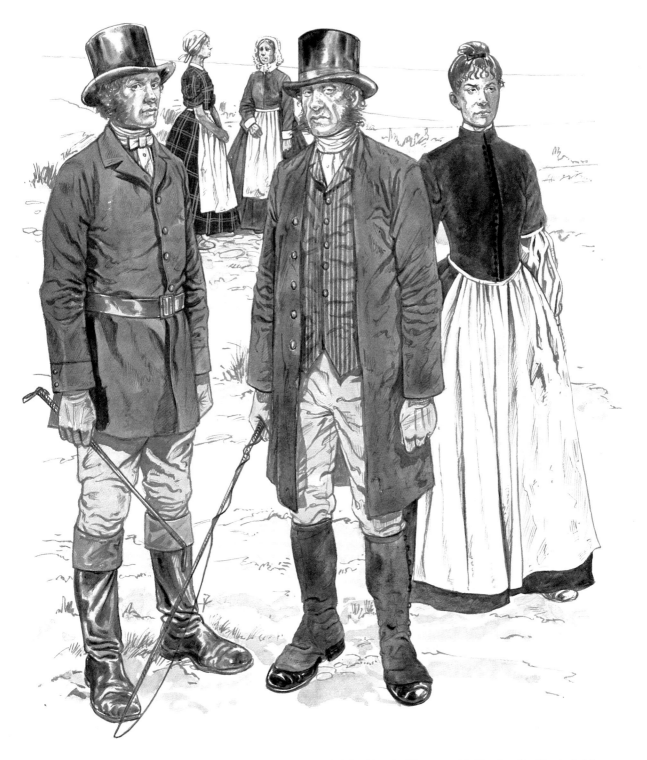

Plate 19 Chapter 7—mid/late 19th century (*Back left*) *Fig. 91* Housemaid (England), (*Back right*) *Fig. 92* Parlourmaid (England), (*Front left*) *Fig. 93* Liveried groom (England), (*Centre front*) *Fig. 94* Liveried coachman (England), (*Front right*) *Fig. 95* Waitress (France).

lar. Elsewhere farm labourers generally wore trousers and braces (*Plate 20, fig. 97*), often with the brace hanging loose on the right hand side to give greater freedom of movement. A scarf was knotted round the neck, serving the dual purpose of supplying warmth in winter and a sweat rag in summer. Additional protective garments were now sometimes supplied by enlightened employers and these included hedger's leather gloves (which had long been in use) and leg pieces, very necessary as most hedges were of thorn. Other protection included armlets of leather for men digging drains, and pieces of crape to cover the faces of those spreading that very corrosive substance—lime.

Agricultural labourers now rarely wore aprons, although an exception was one of leather that contained two pieces of board to protect the stomach and thighs from the pressure of a turf-cutting spade.

Gaiters or leggings were usually worn with breeches, but in their absence wisps of hay or straw were used. Although hardly suitable for country use, chimney-pot hats were widely worn in rural England, as elsewhere, until they were superseded for countrymen by the billycock.

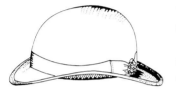

Countryman's billycock hat, 19th century.

The use of natural materials was still widespread in the countryside, hay in particular making a warm lining for boots and wooden-soled shoes, but an unusual form of protection was that worn by some Spanish farming folk who joined layers of wheat, straw or reeds together to make waterproof cloaks and hats. (*Plate 18, fig. 86.*) Leather and sheepskin provided coats and jackets for men like shepherds who had to be out in all weathers, although plaids or blankets were also used. These were either wrapped round the top of the body or folded and carried over the shoulder when not in use. Many shepherds in the UK wore linen smocks treated with linseed oil to make them weatherproof but the increasing use of machinery, in which they were apt to catch, were making them unpopular with other agricultural workers. (*Plate 20, fig. 100.*)

Although there were now few cottage industries, country women still worked in the fields, particularly during haytime and harvest, and in some parts of Europe their clothes had hardly altered for generations. The old corset bodice was still to be seen in rural areas, as well as the sleeveless jacket worn with chemise or blouse. Overskirts, too, continued to be looped up to show the shorter garment below. (*Plate 18, fig. 90.*) In England it was usual for women to discard their gowns when in the fields and to work in their short-sleeved undergarment and petticoat. Sometimes movement was made easier by hitching up the skirts and tying them below the knee, to all intents and purposes providing the wearer if not with trousers at least with a very close approximation to them. As in previous periods bibless aprons served both as a protection and as a means of carrying; some had ties which knotted round the hips as well as the waist, providing, when required, an easily made pouch. Another very effective occupational garment that came into use for summer work in England was the sunbonnet. The wide front brim protected the face from sunburn, something to be avoided at all costs, while the deep flounce at the back prevented sunstroke.

Although fewer women in England worked, even casually, on the land as the century progressed, there were still some in the northern part of the country and in southern Scotland who did so as a full-time occupation. Called 'bondagers' because they were under a bond, or contract, to work for a particular person, they were mostly unmarried and worked in groups with a male labourer who was their overseer. Although at a later date their dress was to be very distinctive, they were mostly notable at this time for dressing alike in short skirts, leather gaiters, heavy boots and sunbonnets.

Women were banned from working underground in English collieries in 1842 but, continuing to work at the pitheads, many kept to the trousers they had found so convenient underground. Trousers were also worn by women colliers in Belgium, though elsewhere female mine workers usually chose ankle-length frocks and coarse pinafores. A simple kerchief was sometimes all that was worn on the head, although many chose to use hats and bonnets which they trimmed in a somewhat pathetic attempt at fashion.

An unusual form of head-gear was part of the dress of the mine-maidens in Cornwall: this consisted of a length of cardboard worn on the top of the head with a flounce of cotton print hanging down the back of the neck. This type of hat gave protection from sun and rain

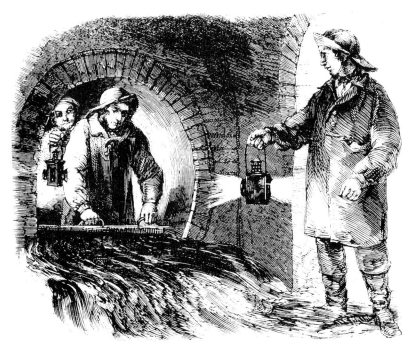

Sewer workers in protective hats, smocks and boots. (From Henry Mayhew *London Labour and the London Poor,* 1851)

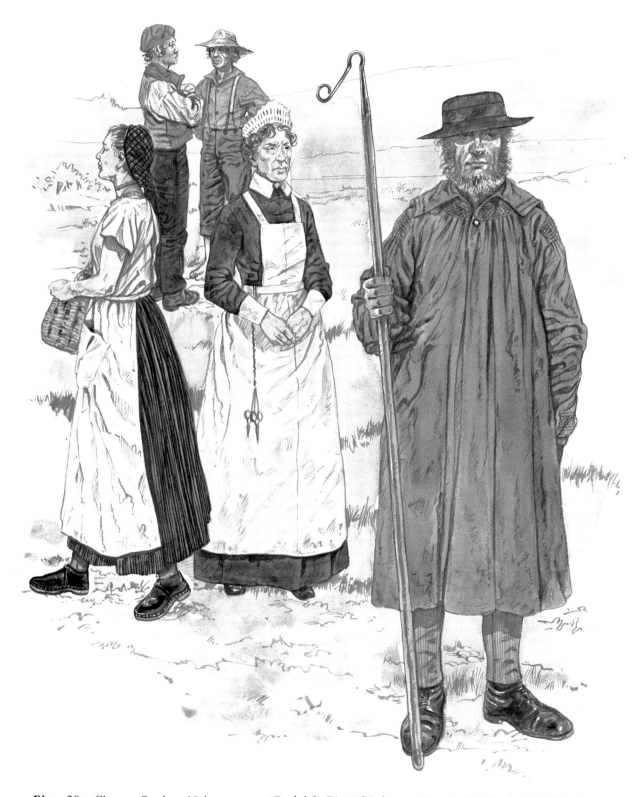

Plate 20 Chapter 7—late 19th century   (*Back left*) *Fig.* 96 Labourer (England), (*Back right*) *Fig.* 97 Rural worker (America), (*Front left*) *Fig.* 98 Factory girl (England), (*Centre front*) *Fig.* 99 Hospital nurse (England), (*Front right*) *Fig. 100* Shepherd (England).

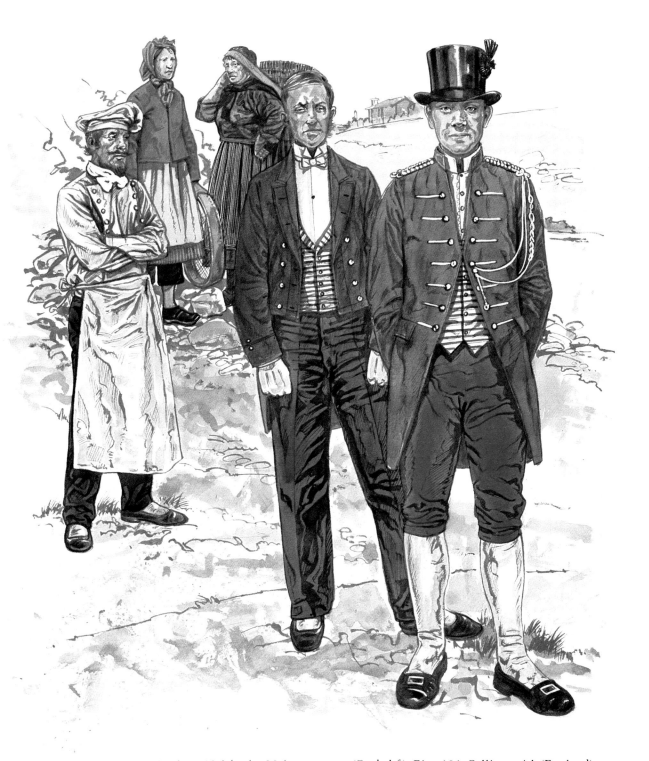

Plate 21 Chapter 8—late 19th/early 20th century (*Back left*) *Fig. 101* Colliery girl (England), (*Back right*) *Fig. 102* Fishwife (Scotland), (*Front left*) *Fig. 103* Chef (France), (*Centre front*) *Fig. 104* Liveried footman—indoor (England), (*Front right*) *Fig. 105* Liveried footman—outdoor (England).

but dust was usually the chief hazard in mining and some girls managed to combat it by wearing a piece of cloth over their face while others used spectacles, or even leather blinkers like those of horses.

Leather was now being widely used by men working underground in an attempt to keep dry, deep fan-tailed hats were combined with capes that covered the shoulders and reached almost to the back of the knees. Various other kinds of hats were also worn, including woollen ones, and sometimes felt hats were coated with clay into which a candle was fixed. Wooden-soled clogs were worn in many mines, those in Lancashire being made in such a way that the feet could be slipped out of them in the event of an accident.

As a rule clothes had to be functional for work in mines, the same was not the case in factories. Totally unsuitable garments like the crinoline, which some employers tried to ban, were fire hazards as well as being liable to catch in machinery, but factory girls continued to try to follow fashion without regard to safety or suitability. However, by the 1870s fashions had changed, skirts had become narrower and the Lancashire mill girl was wearing a back-fastening pinafore over an ankle-length dress. In wooden-soled leather clogs with metal rims and her hair in a net, fashionable as well as functional, she was dressed in clothes well suited to her work. (*Plate 20, fig. 98.*)

A head-covering of some sort was still essential out of doors, although worn less inside. A visitor to England in the 1850s was struck by the fact that even the poorest destitutes found it necessary to have something on their heads, even if only the brim of an old hat. Bonnets

Girls in London's East End match factory wearing aprons over ordinary dress. (The *Graphic*, 1871)

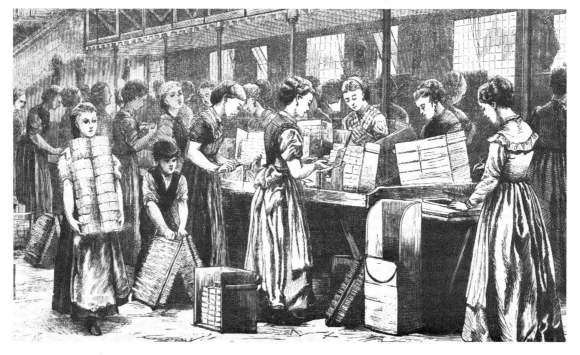

were generally worn by working women; even the dustwomen in their ragged cotton dresses, petticoats and men's jackets, wore the crushed remnants of what might have started life in a fashionable milliners. Many of the clothes of the working people passed from one to another until they were little more than rags. Sometimes, of course, they did not start off as clothes at all for not only was hessian, or burlap, frequently used for coarse aprons but actual sacks, sometimes still with the maker's name, were used as skirts.

Occasionally skirts were dispensed with altogether, as at French seaside resorts where the bathing women, who spent most of the day in the water dipping nervous clients, wore merely a flannel chemise and a kerchief round the head. Bathing women were, of course, barefooted but others doing heavy work like carrying rubbish or coal were obliged to use heavy boots studded with nails.

In France, as in the UK, women undertook many such heavy jobs and there the women porters and carriers of the middle of the century wore calf-length skirts, often red or striped. Their masculine strength was somewhat at variance with the frilly white caps which they put on

Covent Garden porter (centre) wearing a 'porter's knot', or supporting pad, attached to his hat. (1871)

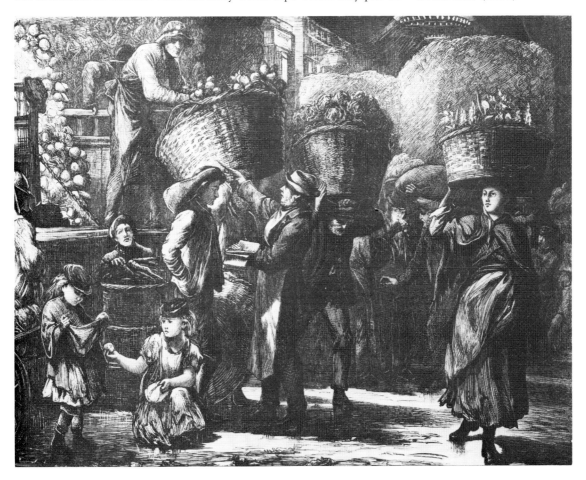

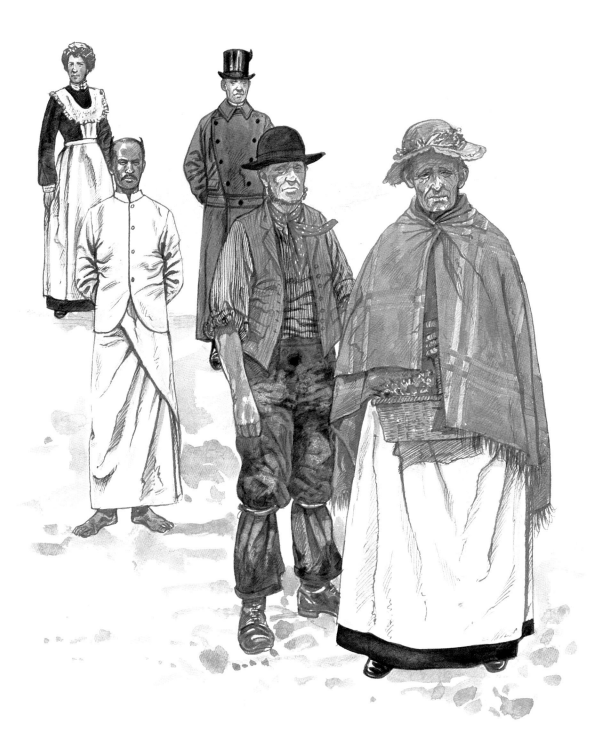

Plate 22 Chapter 8—early 20th century (*Back left*) *Fig. 106* Parlourmaid (England), (*Back right*) *Fig. 107* Chauffeur (England), (*Front left*) *Fig. 108* Yacht steward (British Colonies), (*Centre front*) *Fig. 109* Farm labourer (England), (*Front right*) *Fig. 110* Street trader (England).

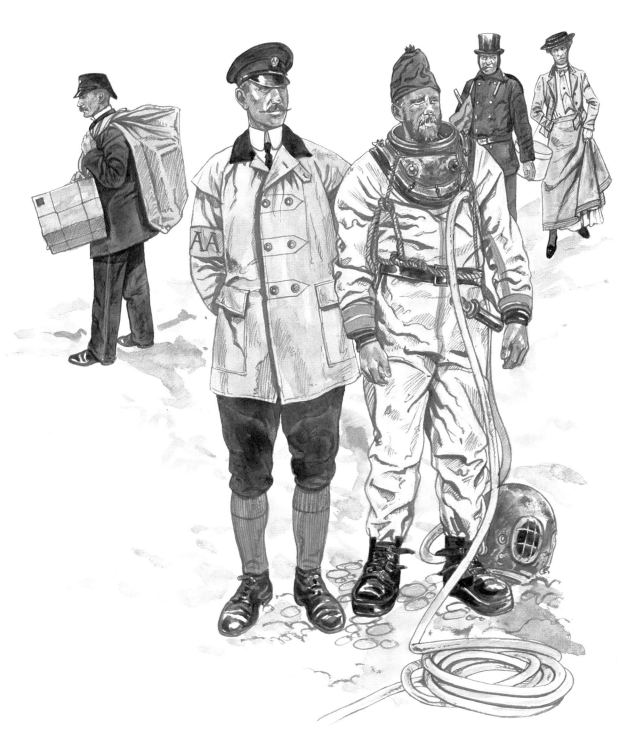

Plate 23   Chapter 8—early 20th century   (*Back left*) *Fig. 111* Postman (England), (*Back centre*) *Fig. 112* Chimney sweep (Germany), (*Back right*) *Fig. 113* Messenger girl (France), (*Front left*) *Fig. 114* Automobile Association patrolman (England), (*Front right*) *Fig. 115* Diver (England).

their heads though, like the male porters in most countries, they wore official badges round their necks. What amounted to a uniform was also worn by the signal women who looked after the level crossings in France for they had black low-crowned hats and blue cloaks.

Railways were the major development of the nineteenth century but, apart from the level crossing ladies, few women were employed by them. Men who worked on the new form of transport at first supplied their own clothes but the companies soon came to see the advantages of a smart uniform. Peaked caps made their appearance about 1848, and a driver, who needed a jacket that buttoned tightly up to the chin, also had a neckerchief and warm trousers. (*Plate 17, fig. 82.*) From an early date guards had considerable status because of their special responsibility and, although their uniforms varied according to the company, they usually wore well-cut frock-coats. (*Plate 17, fig. 83.*)

In addition to the railways there were vast numbers of horse-drawn vehicles for the transport of people and goods. As the number of workers grew, these were increasingly used in the towns. Cab men still wore many-caped overcoats and either top-hats or a predecessor of the bowler hat. They also wore breeches and gaiters, the drivers of horse-drawn trams obtaining even more protection through the use of waterproof aprons which they put over their legs. Although the term 'waterproof' was not used much before the 1880s, a great many different methods were being tried throughout the century to achieve rain-resistant garments. In 1830 Charles Mackintosh introduced a rubberized cloth which, although it was unpopular for a long time on account of its smell, was gradually improved until it became widely used. Waterproofing was also achieved by oiling and tarring leather and various cloths.

One man who might have been glad of a waterproof coat was the butcher whose shop continued, right into the twentieth century, to have an open front. However, he wore instead a particularly heavy type of blue wool cloth made into a double-breasted coat, over which he put a bibless apron of either blue or white. In the early part of the century 'brewers' caps had been popular but like many other tradesmen of the period the butcher soon took to a black top-hat. In some areas both butchers and fishmongers wore smocks.

Most tradesmen and artisans wore aprons of one kind or another. Some, like those of masons, reached right down to the ankles. As a rule these aprons were white, but it was during the nineteenth century that furniture removers and the porters in auction rooms first adopted an apron of green baize.

Although some butchers and fishmongers wore white smocks similar to those of agricultural labourers, hygiene in the food trade had been of comparatively little importance up to now. However, by the middle of the century, bakers and others were beginning to be supplied with white jackets and trousers, and with the flat white caps that were so suitable when trays of bread or biscuits had to be carried on the head.

Although they may have looked quite clean, it is unlikely that hygiene was of much importance to the scores of milkwomen who carried their commodity through the city streets. In the 1850s cows were still sometimes milked at the customers' doors but most of the women carried buckets from dairies. These buckets hung from yokes which, the women claimed, kept them warm in winter. Milkwomen's dresses were short and worn with an apron, a shawl—usually of plaid—a bonnet with a white cap beneath it, and white stockings with boots.

This plaid woollen shawl was for a number of decades to be an indispensable garment for the working class woman who flung it over the head and shoulders whenever she left the house. However, when actually working out of doors, the square shawl was usually folded into a triangle and worn wrapped over shoulders and chest. Crossing sweepers were often women, or young girls, who, being out in all weathers, had to depend entirely upon their shawls for protection. Like the bonnets of most other working women, those of crossing sweepers and street traders often showed an attempt at fashionable trimming. (*Plate 17, figs. 84 and 85.*) Official cleaners (called orderlies) were appointed to clean some London streets in 1843 and were supplied with a uniform of double-breasted jacket and trousers and brimmed hats. These men and the crossing sweepers did much to make life easier for pedestrians but an even more vital service was performed by the public disinfectors who, wearing voluminous white jackets and white trousers, pushed portable ovens in which they fumigated the belongings of those who were suffering from, or had died of, infectious diseases.

Death itself offered a certain amount of employment, for the never-failing funeral business had many conventions including the use of professional mourners (mutes). These were men who accompanied the hearse dressed in coats, trousers, top-hats and gloves of unrelieved black, carrying long staffs or wands. When the funeral was that of an adult a black veil enveloped the hat, a black sash was worn over the left shoulder, and the wand was draped in black. For the funeral of a young girl, or a child, these draperies were white. (*Plate 17, fig. 81.*)

Black was also invariably worn by both male and female shop assistants. In the larger establishments many of these 'lived in' under conditions resembling those of a strict boarding school, including the uniform. For women the attire was a plain, black dress, and for men black frock-coats and trousers. Although neatness was expected, unduly fashionable clothes were frowned upon and might lead to dismissal. White aprons were worn by those working in food shops.

Less control could be exercised over the clothes of clerks, some of whom were now women, and these white-collar jobs were much sought after. Black over-sleeves were usually worn by both sexes, with white

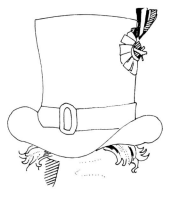

19th-century footman's hat.

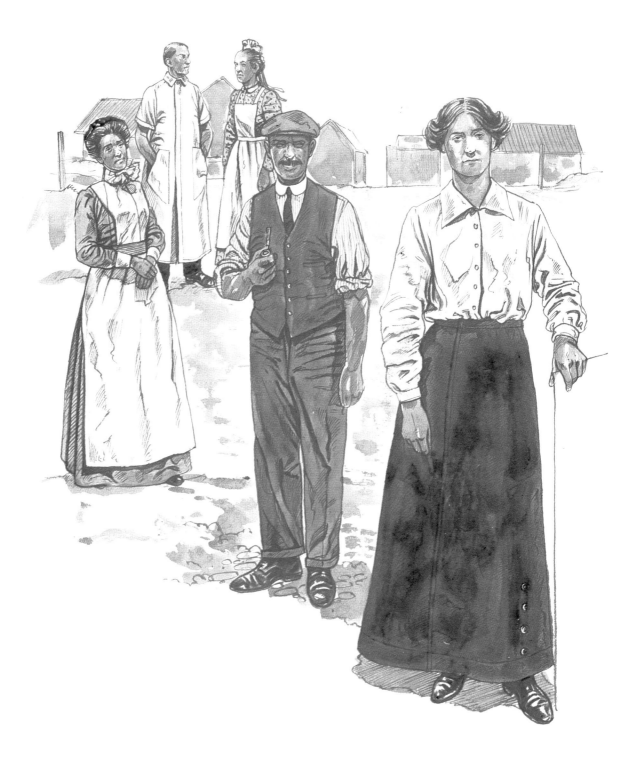

Plate 24 Chapter 8—early 20th century (*Back left*) *Fig. 116* Doctor in theatre coat (England), (*Back right*) *Fig. 117* Housemaid (England), (*Front left*) *Fig. 118* Children's nurse (England), (*Centre front*) *Fig. 119* White collar worker (England), (*Front right*) *Fig. 120* Lady clerk (England).

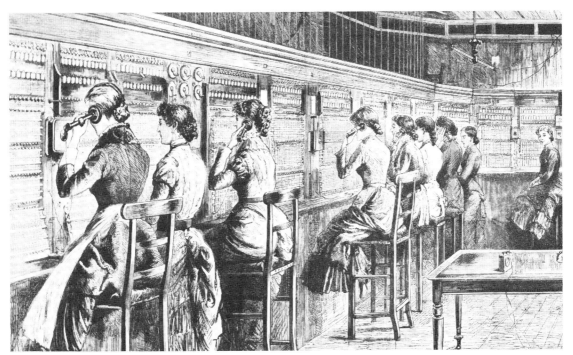

shirts for the men and white collars and cuffs for the women. The over-sleeves were worn to prevent the sleeves of coats and dresses being rubbed and soiled from resting on desks. Some offices laid down rules requiring their employees to dress in clothes of 'a sober nature' and to avoid 'raiment of bright colours'; it is an indication of the conditions under which these people worked that, although the rules forbade the wearing of overshoes and coats, scarves and hats were permitted when the weather was 'inclement'!

Girls at the London Telephone Exchange switchroom and central office. (1833)

In spite of the many new opportunities for employment a great number of people were still in domestic service. The demand for servants was such even in the colonies that many were given assisted passages from Europe.

Due to the more democratic ideas prevalent, the wearing of livery was beginning to be considered a mark of servitude and as time progressed it became increasingly hard to find men who were prepared to wear it. Most of them wished to be like the butler and dress like gentlemen. For some considerable time the butler had worn the clothes of gentlemen of the previous era, tail coat, white waistcoat, breeches, stockings and white gloves. Towards the end of the century he began to follow fashion more closely but wore, as it were, the right clothes at the wrong time. His garb throughout the day was fashionable evening dress of black tail-coat, black trousers, starched white shirt, waistcoat and bow tie. His only departure from formality was in the privacy of the pantry where he discarded his coat and put on a bibbed linen apron. Although the footmen in some houses did dress like the butler, livery

97

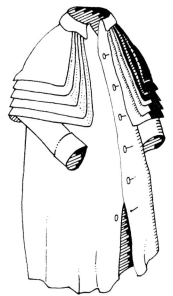

19th-century coachman's box coat.

remained in the larger establishments, as well as in smaller ones, where the newly-rich industrialists ostentatiously put their footmen into magnificent coats and breeches, liberally adorned with braid and buttons. Crested livery buttons were a survival of the days when a serving-man wore his master's insignia upon his back so that he could be distinguished in time of war. In addition to their elaborate clothes, some footmen were expected to wear their hair powdered.

When livery was worn it extended to outdoor servants and dictated the colour of the coachman's caped overcoat or box-coat and the shorter belted coats of grooms. Some coachmen still wore wigs and cocked hats, though the top hat was now more usual. Coachmen wore gaiters and grooms top-boots, while both had chamois gloves and striped waistcoats. (*Plate 19, figs. 93 and 94.*) An important distinction between indoor and outdoor staff was that the stripes on the waistcoats of footmen and other indoor servants were horizontal while those of coachmen and grooms were vertical.

Strangely enough, although livery was slowly disappearing for men, women servants, who up to now had never worn it, were beginning to dress in a uniform style. This may have been partly due to the fact that as fewer men were prepared to enter domestic service women were now doing the more public tasks like waiting at table. Many still provided their own clothes and for a while chose the styles, although those who claimed to have their interests at heart advised them not to choose gay colours or patterns. Nevertheless, when crinolines were at their most popular employers had great difficulty in preventing their maids from wearing them, even when they bumped into whatnots or swept ornaments off tables. Cheap cotton prints were now easily available and by the 1860s it had become customary for a print or plaid dress to be worn in the morning with a bibbed working apron and a cap (*Plate 19, fig. 91*), while in the afternoon a black dress with a more elaborate cap and apron was correct. (*Plate 19, fig. 92.*)

Servants were still expected to go into mourning when some member of their employer's family died and this may have been one of the reasons why lilac and lavender prints were popular for informal wear.

Hotels were now being very efficiently run and the clothes of those who worked in them, and in restaurants, were very similar to what was worn by servants in private houses. For waiters, black jackets and trousers, white shirts and bow ties were worn, sometimes with the addition of a long white bibless apron. Waitresses, according to their means and their places of employment, dressed rather more fashionably than maids, sometimes going without caps and adding protective oversleeves. (*Plate 19, fig. 95.*)

Up to about 1850 nurses and nursery maids were dressed very much like other women servants but after this date in the UK, where there were many large families, they began to assume a position of greater importance. In consequence their clothes became rather more imposing than those of ordinary domestics, though they usually included cap and apron. It was considered a good thing for nursemaids to toss their charges about in their arms and for this reason loose-fitting garments were recommended.

Although the status of women who earned their living was to be greatly improved by the establishment of nursing as a career, nurses at first dressed very much like domestic servants. (*Plate 20, fig. 99.*) As Miss Nightingale herself considered 'washing stuffs' (cottons) to be unsuitable as they required frequent changing, they were not always as practically dressed as servants. The bibbed aprons and caps were like those of maids but their dresses were often of serge and other heavy fabrics. Although hospitals retained their own particular colours and styles, a rigid hierarchy soon developed and a nurse's status was immediately obvious from her uniform.

Strangely enough, although nurses were expected to wear these special clothes, it was still rare for doctors, even when operating, to put anything over their street dress of frock-coats and striped trousers. However, in North America, by 1889, some surgeons were wearing white overalls and jackets, although still with no headcovering or gloves.

Southport, Lancashire lifeboatmen in cork lifejackets. (1886)

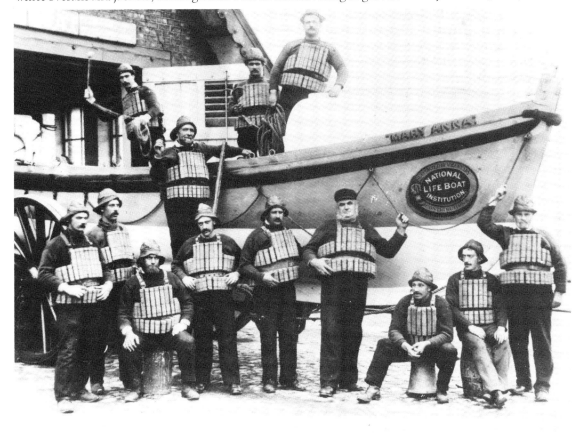

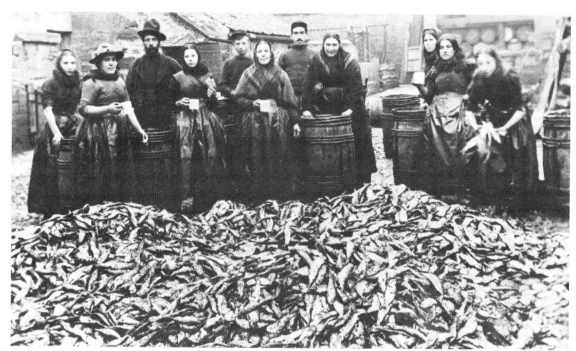

Women herring curers in
Northumberland wearing
protective oilskin aprons.
(1880's)

Fishermen were probably wearing the most advanced types of protective covering: in the Netherlands in the 1850s they had an all-in-one
garment combining boots with what today are called bib-and-brace
overalls or dungarees. Made of oiled leather this was worn with an oiled
leather hat with a deep back brim and oversleeves of the same material.
Few occupational garments can have succeeded in providing such
comprehensive protection. (*Plate 18, fig. 89.*)

Since the early part of the century fishermen in most countries had
been using oiled garments over their blue or grey woollen jerseys and,
although women do not appear to have actually gone to sea, many
engaged either in selling or cleaning fish and wore oilskin aprons or
skirts. Other women who collected bait and fished from the shore
either wore short skirts or trousers, sometimes both together. Different
areas had different styles: in Scotland and parts of France striped skirts
were popular, while Welsh fishergirls favoured red. In parts of the
north of England seamen's jerseys were worn, either with trousers or
skirts tied at the knee to form breeches. In many areas the kerchiefs,
bonnets, or hats which these women wore, had pads on the crowns for
carrying baskets. Where such pads were not worn, the basket was
carried on the back and the weight supported by a band round the
forehead. (*Plate 21, fig. 102.*)

8 Occupational costume in decline

1890–1914

BETWEEN 1890 AND 1914 an era ended and a new way of life began. Although not really apparent until after 1918, distinctions between the leisured and the working classes had begun to blur, while there was a great zeal for reform and an upsurge in democratic ideas.

Social attitudes had their effect upon dress and, as life altered, much of the picturesque quality disappeared from occupational costume, its place being taken by a new practicality and by more protective clothing. As had happened in the case of women servants towards the end of the previous period, uniforms began to take the place of the workers' own clothes; perhaps partly because the increased use of machinery was taking away some of the craftsman's pride in his calling. The tendency towards a greater similarity in dress was encouraged by organizations which saw uniform as useful publicity for themselves and as a possible source of pride and status for the worker.

All railway companies had now put their employees into uniform of some kind, and road transport followed their example. Although up to 1914 the majority of 'carriage folk' remained just that, travelling graciously, if somewhat slowly, behind their own horses, public transport had become essential and quickly took advantage of new methods of locomotion. The internal combustion engine had arrived and its influence in the twentieth century was to be even greater and more far-reaching than that of railways in the nineteenth. At first only a privileged few were involved with the strange new monster but it was not long before the motor car was to affect everyone's lives and provide many new types of employment.

Another factor influencing life at the turn of the century was the improvement in education, particularly in the education of women who now looked for greater freedom and equality; these ambitions led to shorter skirts and simpler styles of dress. Their change in status can be judged by the fact that sixty years from the time when the only respectable career for an educated woman was as a governess, there were 212 doctors, 68,000 nurses, 32,600 teachers and 60,000 women in commercial life in England alone.

Although country ways were not to change a great deal until after 1918, urban life altered considerably. With so many people now living in towns and cities local authorities were becoming more active in taking over the services such as cleaning the streets, and in providing

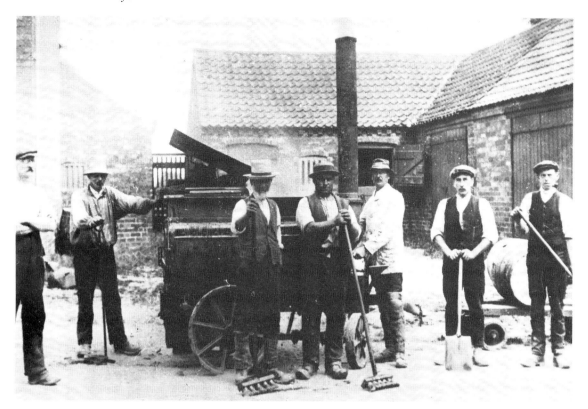

A road-tarring gang in Lincolnshire in 1910. Only two wear anything resembling protective clothing.

amenities. Public health and hygiene increased in importance as the wearing of white coats by many workers from doctors to barbers indicated.

The advent of the bicycle and the popularity it enjoyed in both Europe and America from the end of the nineteenth century had begun a softening-up process in the attitudes previously held towards masculine styles for women—the tailored suit with jacket, skirt and shirt-waister blouse became the business women's uniform.

For men basic garments changed little, apart from the fact that breeches were now rarely seen except in the countryside. Trousers, shirts and waistcoats were universally worn; tie and jacket were added by those in offices and shops. Corduroy was still a favourite fabric for working people although tweed was now widely used and, according to income and status, varying degrees of fine cloth by those who wore suits. A head-covering was still essential and by 1914 the cloth cap was the symbol of the working man, though when he rose from labourer to foreman or supervisor he frequently indicated his superior status by the use of a bowler hat, or derby as it was called in America.

Neckwear had also become an indicator of social position and people in high places wore high, stiff collars. Further down the scale those who had to bend their necks, like clerks and shop assistants, had lower ones while the labourer abandoned the collar completely when at work

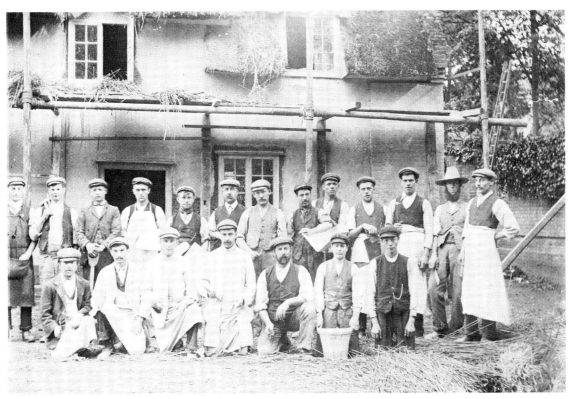

and wore a muffler or neckerchief with his coloured shirt.

Although the billycock hat was still to be seen in rural areas at the turn of the century, it was being replaced by felt hats and cloth caps, with a straw or panama for summer. Both felts and straws were sometimes coated with paint by country people to make them water-proof. Trousers were worn fairly generally but in many ways were not as practical as breeches; leather ties, which were often pieces of harness, had to be strapped on below the knee to help prevent wear and to stop field mice and other small creatures from running up the leg. Gaiters of cloth or leather were used for the same purpose while striped flannel shirts and corduroy waistcoats were the other main garments worn. (*Plate 22, fig. 109.*) Other protective garments for country workers now included a variety of knee pads for thatchers, stone-breakers, harvesters and mole-catchers.

Among country folk a certain prestige was attached to the bowler hat (derby), making it popular with farmers, who sometimes wore breeches to set them apart from their labourers. Bowler hats were also worn as a mark of distinction by the lodge-keepers on many big estates.

Only in very remote areas were homespun fabrics still to be seen, the most usual materials for agricultural workers' trousers being corduroy and tweed, although 'moleskin', the linen and cotton mix with a velvety appearance, was also popular. Most trousers had centre fly-front

English carpenters, painters, thatcher and other building workers at the start of the 20th century. Differences in their dress can be clearly seen.

103

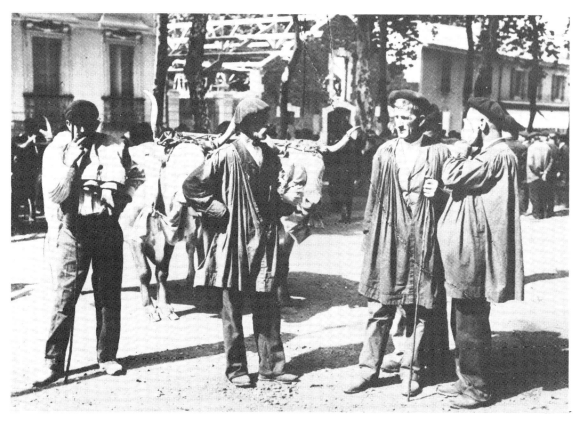

French farmers in smocks and berets, reminiscent of the ancient tunic and cap. (Pre-1914)

fastenings but now and again fall-fronts were used as countrymen still kept their clothes for a very long time and passed them on from one member of the family to another. Sleeved waistcoats, taking the place of jackets which were often too constricting, had a different fabric for the front from that of the back and sleeves. When jackets were worn by such people as gamekeepers they were of plain cotton velvet (velveteen), tweed or corduroy, and often lined for warmth.

In some areas smocks were still in use, though mostly by shepherds and carters and the older men of the community. Feed sacks, with holes cut for head and arms, were a popular (and cheap) form of protection and make an interesting link with one of the oldest of all working garments, the sleeveless tunic.

Large-brimmed hats for protection from the sun were, of course, very much the mark of the agricultural worker in America and the colonies, and cattlemen in Australia fixed corks to the brims to keep off flies. Cowboys, like farm labourers, wore thoroughly practical clothes, a shirt with a neck scarf, used both as a sweat rag and as a dust mask, and denim trousers, or Levis. The latter, called after their originator Levi Strauss, had leather 'chaps' strapped over them protecting the legs from thorns and scrub. A heeled boot helped the cowboy to keep his foot in the stirrup.

Slightly lower-heeled boots, nailed and laced, were general wear for country people including women, a few of whom were still regularly employed on the land. Most of these women wore wide-brimmed hats, though in England the sunbonnet still remained popular.

Although they no longer worked underground, women were still employed at the pitheads of mines and, although few people saw them there, the fact that they wore trousers had long been notorious. As a concession to femininity, short skirts (or rolled-up petticoats) and aprons were worn over the trousers, while padded cotton bonnets and sleeved waistcoats added protection and warmth. On their feet these women wore leather clogs with wooden soles to which irons were attached. (*Plate 21, fig. 101.*)

Men working in the mines usually had blue flannel shirts and corduroy or moleskin trousers, which were tied, like those of farm labourers, below the knee to keep dirt and small pieces of coal from getting up the leg when they were kneeling. Mufflers were worn, and peaked caps with a candle in front although, in place of the candles, lamps were occasionally fixed to straps round the neck. Like the women at the pithead, many miners also wore clogs. When conditions were particularly bad oilskins were used but some work at the coal face was still done naked.

As well as in mines, clogs had long been used by factory workers of both sexes. The typical mill girl's dress at the end of the nineteenth and

Workers in a German sausage factory each wearing two aprons in addition to an overall. (Pre-1914)

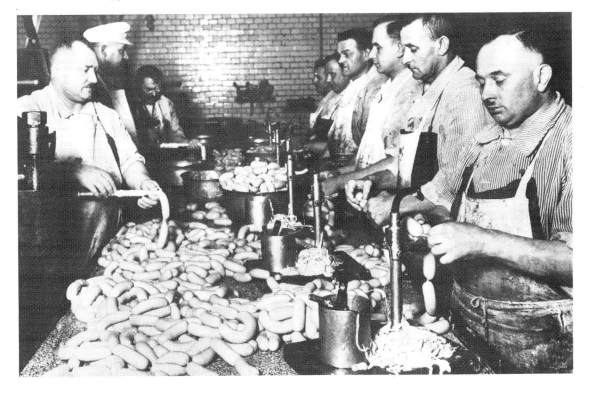

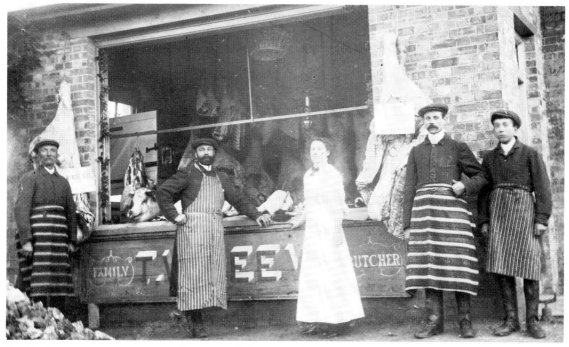

Staff of an English
butcher's shop wearing
both horizontally and
vertically striped aprons.
(Early 20th century)

the start of the twentieth centuries included these clogs and a plaid
shawl. Factories processing food, however, had begun to give some
thought to hygiene and to introduce overalls. These had the advantage
not only of protecting the product but also of enabling the workers to
wear their better, instead of their oldest, clothes during working hours.

Many white-collar workers removed their jackets and worked in
their shirtsleeves (*Plate 24. fig. 119*), craftsmen did the same but
usually added a white, bibbed apron.

Occupational aprons still varied. Sometimes the fabric used had
obvious practical application, such as the leather ones that protected
blacksmiths from sparks; the reason for others was more obscure. Green
baize, for instance, was possibly used by furniture removers because it
was soft and suitable for polishing.

A blue-and-white-striped apron was now usual for butchers, replacing the older plain blue one. Occasionally white ones were worn for
serving customers and these had no bibs, while the striped ones had
and were held in place with a loop round the neck. Up to 1914 most
butchers' shops had open fronts and master butchers still wore heavy,
knee-length coats of blue cloth (which did not stain easily) with a
fly-front covering the buttons. The straw boater which came into use
about this time is believed to have been used originally to provide
protection from the blood that dripped from hanging joints.

Leather aprons, leg shields and wooden-soled boots still protected
slaughtermen while men who carried meat in the markets had long
overalls of white or blue linen.

Bakers, who had frequently in the past chosen white garments as a form of inverted camouflage, were now thinking of them in terms of hygiene and began to use white aprons with white jackets and caps. In very large bakeries white trousers were worn as well.

Most shopkeepers' aprons were without bibs and reached the ankles at this time, though assistants in drapery shops did not use them at all. Their jobs depended to a great extent upon being able to maintain spotless collars and cuffs. Assistants in shoe shops, however, did wear white aprons as they had to take customers' feet on their laps.

Fewer commodities were now hawked in the street and milk and letters were delivered to the door. Milk roundsmen were very smart, pushing small trolleys and wearing blue or white jackets with top-hats or bowlers, though these soon began to be replaced by peaked caps. Postmen's uniforms in the UK had been blue since 1861, their scarlet piping being all that remained of the original royal red livery. From 1896 to about 1910 their caps were of a style used by postmen in France with peaks protecting both face and neck. (*Plate 23, fig. 111.*)

In the days before advertizing, occupational costume had been an easily understood means of communication and chimney sweeps were still recognizable, even when they were clean, by their top-hats. (*Plate 23, fig. 112.*) Of the other street characters still to be seen the most common were now the flower and fruit women in their straw hats and plaid shawls. (*Plate 22, fig. 110.*) These shawls were so much a part of the street trader for generations that in Ireland right up to the middle of the present century women who sold goods from baskets or barrows were invariably known as 'shawlies'.

City streets were now, of course, a great deal more congested and, though most of the traffic was still horse drawn, the occasional motor car had begun to make its appearance. Originally the drivers of horse-drawn buses and trams had adopted the dress of private coachmen but now usually had thick serge jackets, breeches, gaiters and boots with a leather apron that reached from feet to armpits. This apron served a double purpose by protecting them from the weather as well as from the mud and dirt thrown up by the horses. Brown bowler hats were worn by some drivers though top-hats remained popular. For additional protection large umbrellas were attached to the bus behind the driver's back.

The conductors on public transport usually wore trousers rather than breeches, with bowler hats in winter and straw boaters in summer until, eventually, peaked caps were introduced. When electric trams and motor buses made their appearance, leather aprons were no longer necessary and were replaced with heavy coats or mackintoshes. Goggles of either plain or tinted glass were also supplied and remained essential as long as vehicles had open fronts.

Following the example of the first drivers of public transport

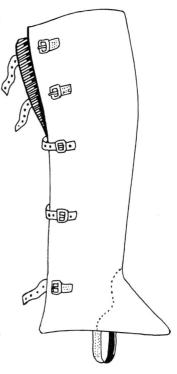

Slaughterman's leg shield, late 19th/early 20th century.

vehicles, the earliest drivers of motor-taxicabs also adopted the style of dress used by their opposite numbers in private service, close-fitting jackets, breeches and gaiters.

As more and more people began to have 'motors' it became increasingly difficult to acquire, as had originally been done, the driver with the car. For this reason early motoring magazines exhorted their readers to 'get your coachman taught to drive at once'. Whether it was the coachman or some other member of staff who eventually took the wheel, the tradition of driver and footman sitting side by side in livery coats and breeches continued, footmen riding on the motor cars as they had done on the coaches, with warm rugs round their knees. One type of chauffeur's livery consisted of coat and breeches with a detachable apron or skirt of the same fabric which, when fastened round the waist, gave the appearance of an overcoat. (*Plate 22, fig. 107.*) However, most chauffeurs wore double-breasted jackets with two rows of buttons from shoulder to hem and breeches without the skirts. Goggles and peaked caps soon replaced top-hats that, it was found, blew off at high speeds. For bad weather cream-coloured oilskin coats were provided. In 1909 short oilskin jackets were worn by the road scouts of the new Automobile Association, peaked caps and arm bands were also issued to these men, although they had to provide their own stockings, shoes and breeches. (*Plate 23, fig. 114.*)

A form of overall had already been used in some factories, buttoning down the front for men and down the back for women, but trousered overalls were only now beginning to make their appearance. It was not long, however, before the bib-and-brace overall became associated with engines, its comprehensive nature making it particularly suitable for use when bending over machinery. The heavy cotton of which these garments were made—dungaree—eventually gave its name to the garment.

Although it was becoming more difficult to find domestic staff, there were still some very large establishments where footmen dressed as elaborately as before and where a 'matching set' of footmen were highly prized. In such places there were usually several types of livery, for informal, formal and state occasions. Informal livery usually consisted of trousers and tailcoats while the more formal styles were the eighteenth century ones of ornamented coats, breeches and silk stockings and even powdered hair, white cotton gloves being worn both indoors and out. (*Plate 21, figs. 104 and 105.*) Overcoats reaching the ankles were fashionable for head footmen and extremely practical as their work often required them to wait for long periods out-of-doors.

In spite of the fact that women servants were all dressed much alike and wore certain types of apron and cap according to status, they had never worn livery and now never would. Matching striped, spotted or plain cotton dresses were worn, (*Plate 24, fig. 117*) though not always

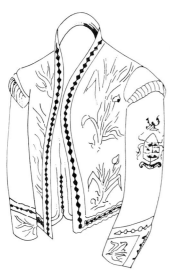

Postillion's jacket, 19th and 20th centuries.

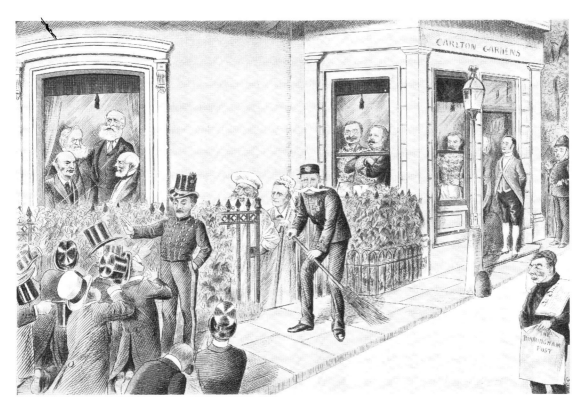

provided for morning work, with large white aprons and caps changed in the afternoon for black dresses and fancy caps and aprons. (*Plate 22, fig. 106.*) In North America, where it was becoming increasingly hard to get people to enter service, the cap was beginning to be considered the mark of servitude and was often dispensed with altogether.

In private houses, restaurants and clubs all chefs now had white double-breasted jackets fastened with two rows of buttons. Their white hats were somewhat taller than before and a white bibless apron was put on over the jacket, with a white handkerchief or sweat rag round the neck. (*Plate 21, fig. 103.*)

Staff in clubs dressed similarly to the staff of private houses with footmen in livery and waiters in black tail-coats, trousers, white shirts and bow ties. Page boys, much in demand in clubs though seldom to be found in private establishments, had tightly-fitting jackets and matching trousers. Some clubs dressed their men servants like ships' stewards in plain white linen jackets and dark trousers. When the staff on privately-owned yachts came from countries in the East, these white jackets were worn over national costume. (*Plate 22, fig. 108.*)

Children's nurses had been part of many households for centuries and their clothes similar to those of other women servants. However, their status began to alter about the middle of the nineteenth century and they adopted the plain dark dress of housekeepers. When nursing

Cartoon showing public figures as club servants. (*Truth* Christmas Number, 1892)

began to be recognized as a profession they changed to the type of garments worn by senior nurses in hospitals, usually wearing grey dresses in winter and white in summer, always with large white aprons. Indoors an elaborate cap was worn and out of doors a bonnet, often with streamers. (*Plate 24, fig. 118.*) Following the establishment of training colleges at the end of the nineteenth century many 'nannies' who had not been trained in them nevertheless copied their uniforms.

Although fisherwomen and girls cannot be said to have worn uniforms at any time, there had always been considerable uniformity in both their working dress and their Sunday, or festive, attire. For work, trousers were now less common and the working day was usually spent in coarse cotton blouses, calf-length flannel skirts (often striped), and striped flannel aprons, with either a shawl or a heavy coat put round the shoulders for warmth. Stockings, when worn for work, were usually black, though white ones appeared for Sundays. Baskets were still carried on the head or on the shoulders with a supporting band round the brow. When sorting or preparing fish for market, black oilskin skirts or bibbed aprons were worn. Men also wore waterproof aprons for this purpose, and at sea oilskin coats, usually without buttons which tended to catch in the nets.

Since the eighteenth century diving suits had developed in several different ways. Watertight rubber garments with metal helmets now enabled divers to remain safely under water for long periods. By the end of the century these suits were of solid sheet india rubber or heavy, rubberized white cotton. Copper and brass helmets had glass windows through which the diver could see and tubes in the helmet reached the surface providing him with air. A woollen cap was usually put on under the helmet and, as with other clothing under the suit, prevented friction. Heavy, leather boots were used, the wooden soles of which were weighted with lead. (*Plate 23, fig. 115.*)

In their new business life women's tailored coats, skirts and blouses gave an impression of efficiency. (*Plate 23, fig. 111 and Plate 24, fig. 120.*) Among the professions into which they had eventually succeeded in breaking was that of medicine where, at about the same time, a specific working dress was beginning to appear. By the turn of the century many doctors were wearing washable white linen coats, or jackets, and the former were also worn by women, the only difference being that theirs buttoned from right to left instead of the traditional masculine way. (*Plate 24, fig. 116.*) White linen caps and masks were now being used in the operating theatre, while rubber gloves were introduced during the last decade of the nineteenth century. These were originally considered as a protection for the hands rather than as a means of protecting the patient from infection, for the doctor who invented them only did so from a wish to spare the fair hands of his theatre sister, whom he later married, from the effects of carbolic acid!

9 War and women in trousers

1914–1925

CHANGES WERE ALREADY ON THE WAY before the 1914–18 War but it, and its consequences, hastened the end of a society in which some people worked while others did not. By 1939 most men, and many women, had paid occupations of some kind, although in the years between the two wars there were never enough jobs to go round.

Since early times there had been a distinction, sometimes slight, between working dress and Sunday, or festive, dress. Now, because all but the very poor had more garments in their wardrobes, the difference was becoming less obvious and occupational clothes were either a protective covering or a uniform to be discarded as soon as work was finished.

Uniforms had come about originally as a means of identification but had subsequently been provided to encourage smartness—always good for the image of an organisation—and a sense of belonging. Protective garments, on the other hand, were either a safety measure or a means of keeping clean. Uniform had always been supplied by the employer, even if only on loan or hire, but protective clothes, having originated from the ingenuity of the worker and, up to the War years, usually provided by him, tended to be his own property.

However, it was not only the War, leveller though it was, that changed attitudes to work and working clothes for, between 1914 and 1925, socialism was spreading throughout Europe and the movement towards greater equality and better conditions was gathering momentum.

Part of the socialist ideal was to prevent people being at risk in the course of their work, and this was eventually to lead to various statutory regulations. Nevertheless, though machinery was becoming more complicated and dangerous it was some time before adequate protection was forthcoming. Even when it was available it was frequently not used through conservatism and a wish not to be thought weak and fearful. On account of this, men's basic working dress for some time remained shirt, sleeveless waistcoat, trousers and cap. The shirt was now usually coloured, striped or checked, with a coloured collar, which in North America was often attached, though still separate in the UK where the collarless shirt was worn for work and often covered with a muffler, either crossed over the chest inside the waistcoat, or worn hanging straight down from the throat. The trousers were kept in place with braces (called suspenders in North America), though these were usually hidden by the waistcoat. When a belt was worn, the buckle was frequently twisted round to the back to prevent it catching on anything. The cloth cap was also sometimes reversed to allow the peak to protect the back of the neck. Only in a few instances, such as mining, did men work in trousers alone for in England, until comparatively recent times, it was considered that only 'the gentry' could demean themselves by being seen bare to the waist.

Most working women wore skirt and blouse with apron or overall, while shawls had been discarded in favour of coats and jackets. Generally, women wore shoes but many men still had hob-nailed boots. Rubber Wellington boots were becoming common when work was wet or muddy.

In the early 'twenties many workers who needed particularly strong clothes for heavy work, such as on building sites, wore army surplus trousers, jackets and boots.

Occupational dress varied little in Europe and North America, though one or two specifically national garments remained, such as the loose blue blouses used in France and Belgium.

The motor car had now begun to assume a place of considerable importance in the world. The first drive-in petrol and service station opened in Pittsburgh in 1913 while in England the first off-the-road petrol pump was installed in 1916. Bib-and-brace overalls and boiler suits had arrived in England from North America during the early years of the century and were now worn by the mechanics and 'motor engineers' who worked at the petrol pumps and service stations. (*Plate 25, figs. 124, 125.*) The fabrics were denim and dungaree and separate oversleeves were also used.

Chauffeurs still dressed in jacket, breeches and boots, or gaiters, though now with a peaked cap, as the top-hat had been discarded. (*Plate 25, fig. 123.*) Leather coats were sometimes used but were less common. In very cold weather a heavy overcoat liberally endowed with livery buttons was worn and for maintenance work in the garage a cleaning coat. (*Plate 25, figs. 121 & 125.*) Cuffs on livery coats and jackets were narrow as wide ones were liable to catch on door handles when the chauffeur helped his passengers in and out of the car. Leather gloves were always worn and were usually brown.

Soon after the outbreak of war it became obvious that women were going to have to take over a great many jobs that had previously been done by men. As a result, thousands of them began to do work that they had never been permitted to do before, and which they would cease doing as soon as the national emergency was over. However, the fact that they had done these jobs, even if only for a short time, had a tremendous effect upon dress and did away with many conventions that had previously restricted women. Hemlines rose, hair was cut short

112

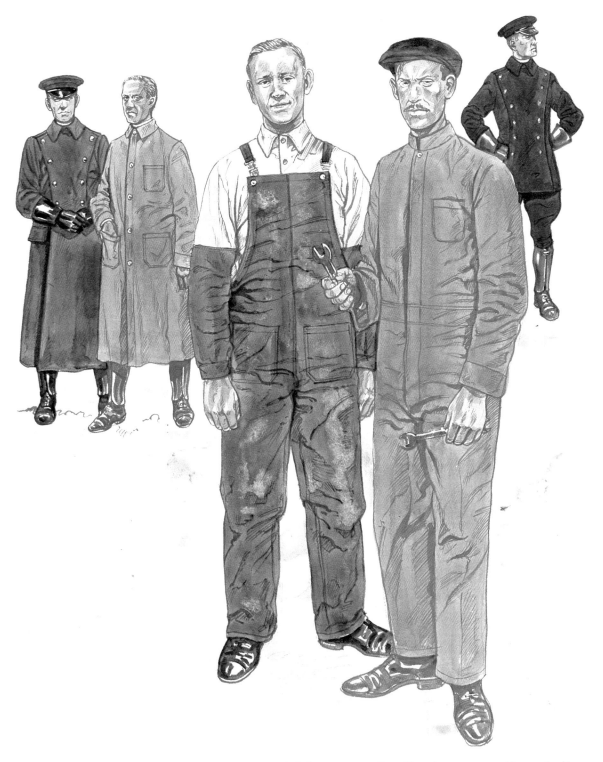

Plate 25 Chapter 9—c. 1914—England (*Back left*) *Fig. 121* Chauffeur in overcoat, (*Centre back*) *Fig. 122* Chauffeur in cleaning coat, (*Back right*) *Fig. 123* Chauffeur in jacket and breeches, (*Front left*) *Fig. 124* Motor mechanic, (*Front right*) *Fig. 125* Motor engineer.

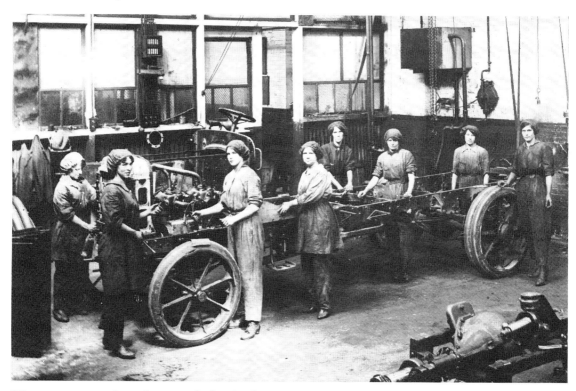

Women war workers in engineering shop in overalls and boiler suits. (1917)

and, for the first time in the Western world, trousers became acceptable female attire.

Numerous English women, 700,000 by 1917, were employed in making munitions and the use of protective clothing for health and safety at work was, almost for the first time, given serious consideration. Although the efforts made were not always successful, workers in some factories were known as Lloyd George's canaries because not only their clothes but their skins turned yellow from chemicals. Nevertheless, a great deal was done to prevent such happenings. Linen trousers and overalls or jackets, rubber boots and close-fitting caps were issued (*Plate 26, fig. 126*) with goggles, rubber gloves and fireproof overalls for particularly dangerous jobs. Trousers were, of course, ideal because not only did they give freedom of movement but they offered protection from high explosive powder and did not catch in machinery as skirts would have done.

Up to now women of all classes had kept their hair long, but in some munition works there was a likelihood of being scalped by hair catching in machinery, so not even a wisp was permitted to show. Confining their long tresses under caps presented many women with problems and they cut their hair short. The new freedom this gave encouraged them to retain short hair after the War and gave rise to the bobs and shingles of the 'twenties.

Other women went to work as agricultural labourers, or land girls,

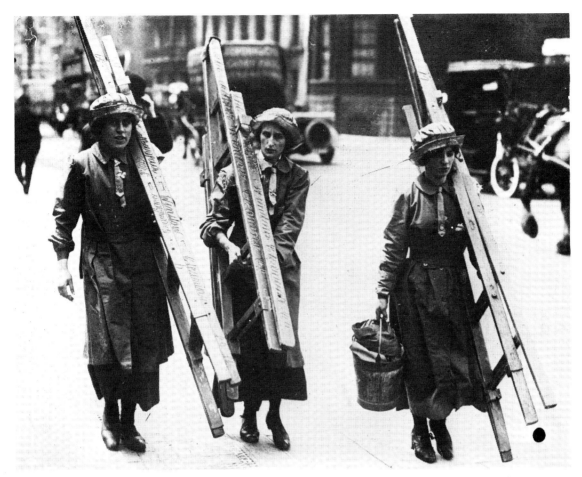

and here again skirts were inappropriate. Instead, breeches were provided with linen overalls, gaiters and boots, or, for stock work, clogs.
Wide-brimmed hats were also issued (*Plate 26, fig. 127*), and a
mackintosh for bad weather. The linen overalls of the women in both
these occupations were generally khaki or beige, though the effects of
washing produced quite a variety of colour.

The railways, tramways and bus companies, as well as the postal
service, called upon women for help and, in most cases, the clothes
with which they were issued were similar to the uniforms of the men
whose jobs they had taken over. However, they were usually given the
option of a skirt if they did not wish to wear trousers.

Uniforms were not always immediately forthcoming and some
women who worked for the post office wore their own blouses, skirts
and straw hats with only an arm band for identification. (*Plate 26, fig.
129.*) Bus conductresses' uniforms varied according to which company
they worked for, those with the London General Omnibus Company
wearing navy jackets and skirts with white piping, and a matching hat
with a badge. (*Plate 26, fig. 128.*)

Women belonging to a
firm of London window
cleaners wearing
uniforms. (1914-18)

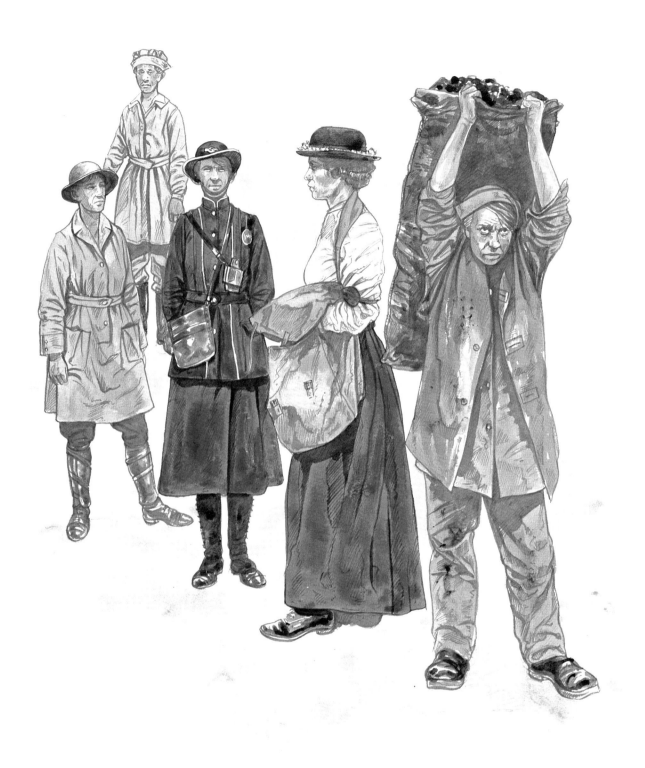

Plate 26 Chapter 9—1914-1918—England (*Back left*) *Fig. 126* Munitions worker, (*Front left to right*) *Fig. 127* Land-girl, *Fig. 128* Bus conductress, *Fig. 129* Post woman, *Fig. 130* Woman coal carrier.

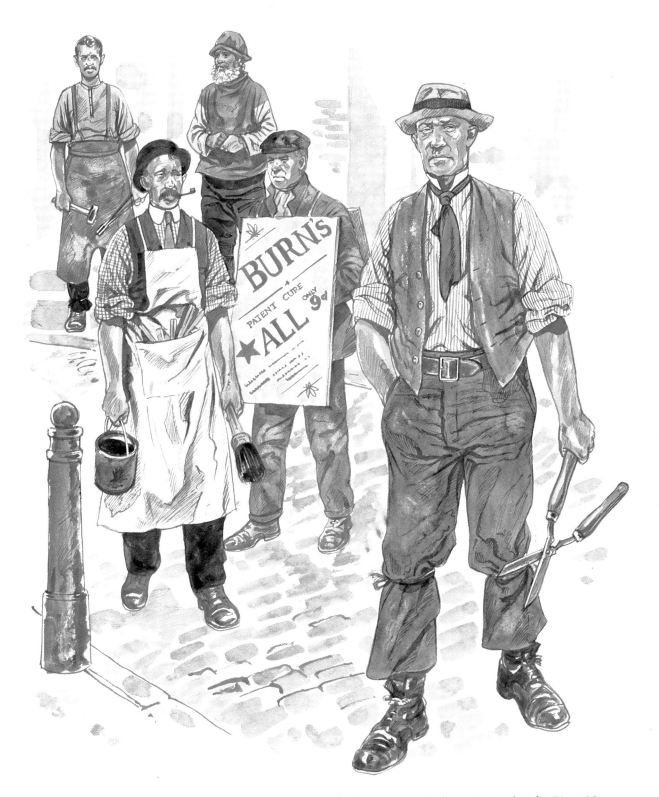

Plate 27 Chapter 9—early 1920's—England (*Back left*) *Fig. 131* Blacksmith, (*Back right*) *Fig. 132* Sea fisherman, (*Front left*) *Fig. 133* Housepainter, (*Centre front*) *Fig. 134* Sandwich-board man, (*Front right*) *Fig. 135* Gardener Handyman.

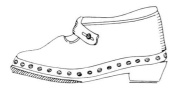

Wooden-soled shoe, or clog. 20th century.

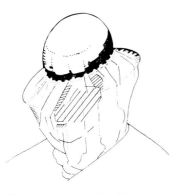

Beekeeper's veiled hat, 20th century.

Many labouring jobs, such as tarring the streets, sweeping chimneys and carrying coal, were also done by women during the war years. Overalls and trousers again being usual. (*Plate 26, fig. 130.*)

When peace returned most women, some no doubt thankfully, but others reluctantly, gave up their jobs and returned to their homes. But as so many men had been killed there was a tremendous surplus of unmarried women for whom a career seemed the only future, though the unemployment that came with the recession of the post-war years meant that there were fewer opportunities for them.

One field in which women did continue to work was nursing. All hospital nurses, and many children's nannies, were now in uniforms that were both practical and hygienic with short skirts and less elaborate headgear. Since training colleges had been set up for them, children's nannies had begun to assume quite a different status and were no longer looked upon as upper servants. Because of this improvement in their standing, some of the unqualified ones copied the uniforms of hospital nurses until a stop was put to it in 1919 when the nursing profession obtained legal professional status in England.

A complaint that seems to have been general among nurses and nannies of the period was that the uniforms, though practical, were cold, which goes to show that, even when a lot of thought has been given to them, specially designed occupational uniforms are not always entirely suited to the job.

One occupational costume that had long been suited to work, the smock, had now almost completely disappeared because of changing conditions. The increased use of tractors and other farm machinery made a loose, voluminous garment of this kind a hazard rather than a help and few countrymen, apart from shepherds, now wore it for work. Even shepherds had dispensed with it by the 1920s. The shepherds themselves were fast disappearing and those that were left wore fleecy white coats with capes, specially made with hand-sewn, saddle-stitched seams to keep out the wet, or, if they could not afford these, whatever assortment of clothing they could gather. Heavy boots and leather leggings, with additional pieces of leather worn on top of the laces, protected legs and ankles. Corduroy was sometimes used for gaiters as well as for trousers and jackets. In some areas shepherds had large umbrellas which they carried strapped across their backs. It is interesting to note that however well wrapped up a shepherd might be, neck and throat were usually bare.

On some of the larger and more progressive farms the new emphasis on hygiene brought about the use of white overalls and caps for milking and dairy work.

In spite of the increasing use of overalls among other occupations, miners still had no distinctive dress, wearing whatever old jackets and trousers they had, usually with the addition of a cloth cap and a woollen muffler. There were, as yet, few pit-head baths or changing rooms and clothes had to be dried out in front of coal fires in the miners' homes. Underground, depending upon the work, trousers were often the only garment, though 'drawers' resembling the bottom part of pyjamas, might be worn. Shirts were frequently discarded and used only to wipe off sweat. Wooden-soled leather clogs, being an efficient means of keeping the feet dry and avoiding slipping, were still worn, though many miners now had laced boots. Cloth caps were the usual head-gear. When mechanical coal cutters were introduced it was found necessary to wear protective knee pads once again.

In most factories men and women wore ordinary working dress, though overseers and foremen might wear suits and bowler hats, for the bowler hat was still a status symbol. Skilled workers usually kept on collar and tie, though jackets were dispensed with and replaced with a

Brewer's draymen (in aprons and caps) making a delivery to a public house. (Pre-1914)

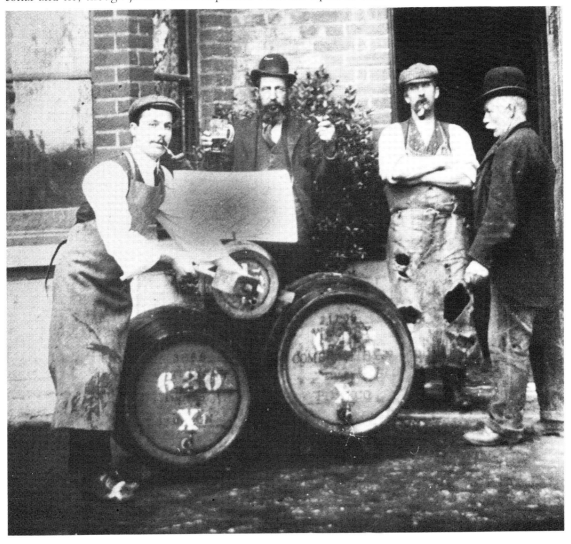

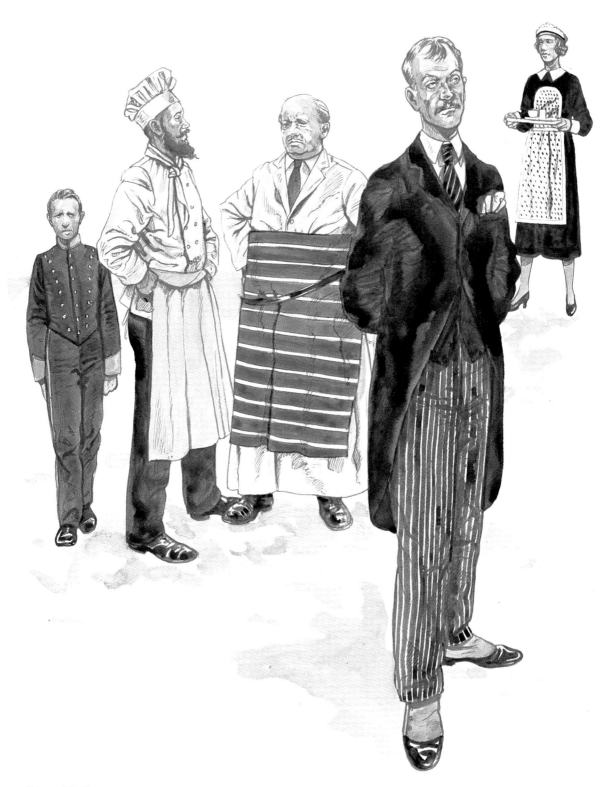

Plate 28 Chapter 9—early 1920's—England (*Back right*) *Fig. 136* Parlour-maid, (*Centre left to right*) *Fig. 137* Page boy, *Fig. 138* Chef, *Fig. 139* Butcher, (*Front right*) *Fig. 140* Department store floorwalker.

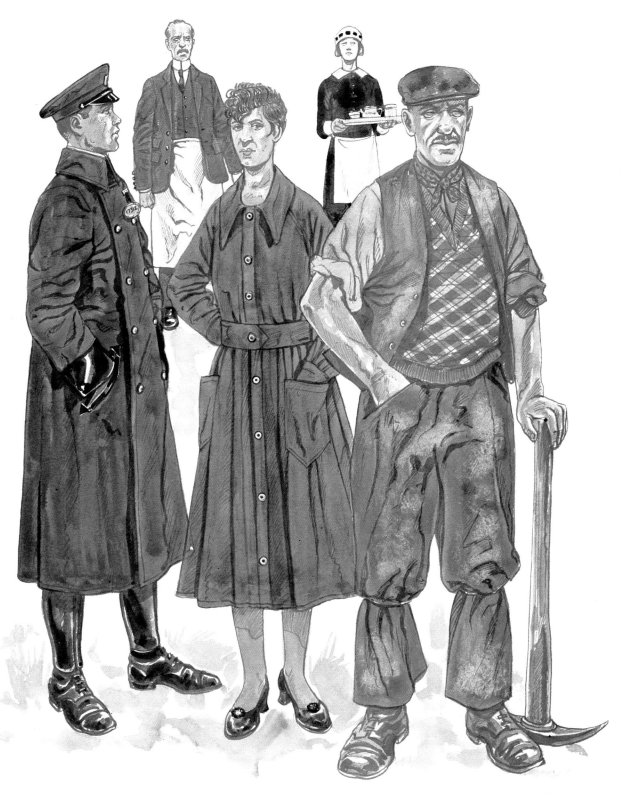

Plate 29   Chapter 10—late 1920's—England   (*Back left*) *Fig. 141* Grocer/Greengrocer, (*Back right*) *Fig. 142* Waitress, (*Front left*) *Fig. 143* Commercial driver, (*Centre front*) *Fig. 144* Office worker, (*Front right*) *Fig. 145* Navvy.

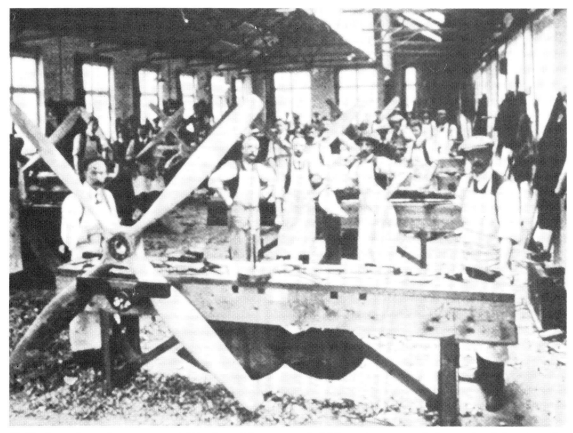

Skilled workers in a British aircraft factory, with bibbed white carpenters' aprons over ordinary working clothes. (c.1914)

bibbed working apron held by a loop round the neck. (*Plate 27, fig. 133.*) Women's aprons usually had no bibs though for some of the more unpleasant and messy jobs, such as gut scraping and tripe-dressing, waterproof overalls were beginning to be supplied.

Short white overall jackets were now the usual wear of many white-collar workers such as barbers, barmen and shopkeepers. Grocers and butchers used them and added an apron. (*Plate 28, fig. 139.*) Where food was not involved, or a hygienic appearance unnecessary, shopkeepers and their assistants preferred brown drill coat overalls. Assistants in drapery shops still wore black suits, white shirts and dark ties.

Many shops had taken on female assistants for the first time during the War and in grocery shops they wore white pinafores or overalls. In large city drapery stores, where they had long been employed, some were now provided with coloured dresses made in current styles, and for those who had taken over the jobs of male commissionaires there were matching cloaks to keep them warm. Generally speaking, however, drapery assistants' plain black dresses with white collars and cuffs were their own property. In very high-class fashion houses fitters were expected to wear white gloves while attending to important clients.

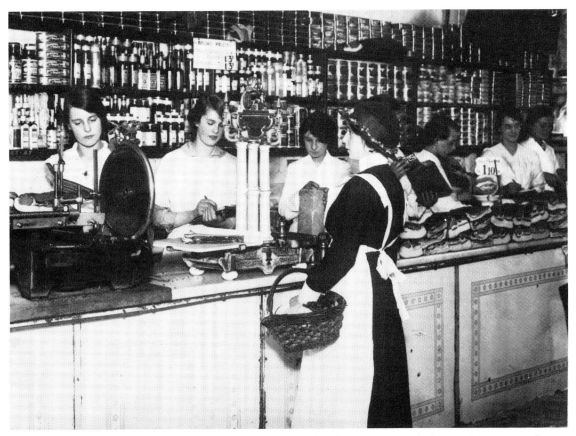

Managers and floor walkers were formally dressed in black morning-coats, black waistcoats and striped trousers. (*Plate 28, fig. 140.*) With a white shirt, dark tie, and black shoes, this was the usual wear of the city business man of the period.

There were not many street traders to be seen now, apart from the flower girls with their large baskets and plaid shawls, though the ice-cream vendor on his bicycle had become a familiar sight. He wore a short white jacket over ordinary working clothes, and either a cloth cap or a white one with a peak.

Although his boards can hardly be described as costume, the publicity element of something worn reached its climax in the sandwich man (*Plate 27, fig. 134*). In spite of not being engaged himself in what he advertised, he was a direct descendant from the street characters of the seventeenth century who had carried flags or banners announcing they were rat catchers. Under his boards, the sandwich man wore ordinary dress and, usually, a cloth cap.

Cloth caps were nearly always a part of the working man's costume but peaked caps accompanied uniform. Most public service uniforms comprised navy blue jackets and trousers, though railway porters were among the few to retain the nineteenth-century sleeved waistcoat.

A domestic servant, hat especially donned for shopping, is served by overalled assistants in a London grocery.

123

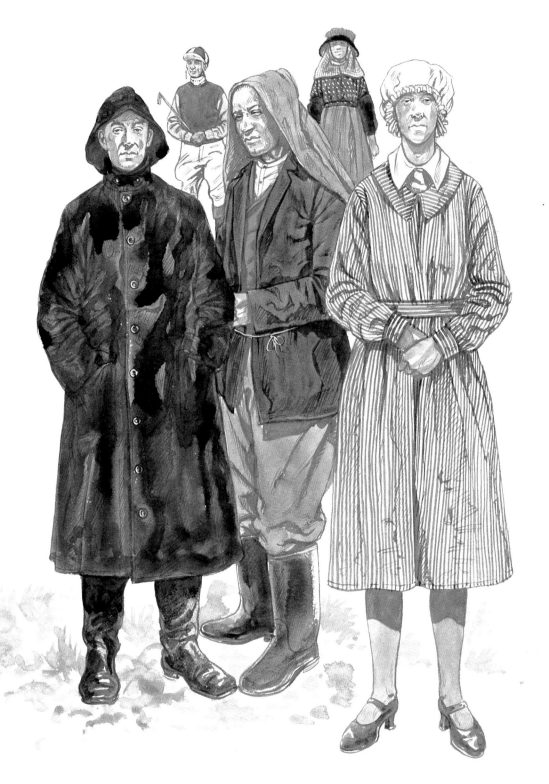

Plate 30 Chapter 10—early 1930's—England (Back left) *Fig. 146* Jockey, (*Back right*) *Fig. 147* Bondager (Fieldworker, Scotland), (*Front left*) *Fig. 148* Ship's pilot, (*Centre front*) *Fig. 149* Farm labourer, (*Front right*) *Fig. 150* Factory worker.

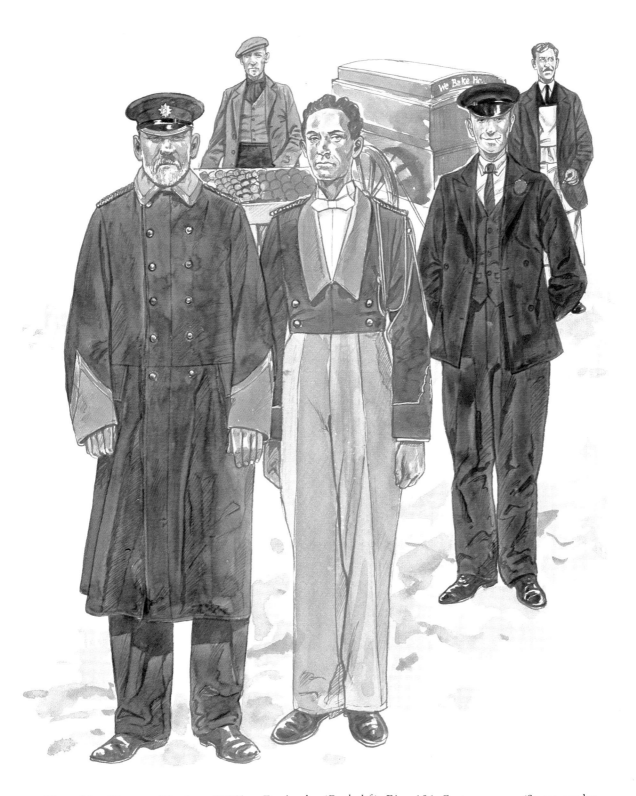

Plate 31 Chapter 10—late 1930's—England (*Back left*) *Fig. 151* Costermonger (Street trader, London), (*Back right*) *Fig. 152* Baker's deliveryman, (*Front left*) *Fig. 153* Cinema commissionaire, (*Centre front*) *Fig. 154* Cinema usher, (*Front right*) *Fig. 155* Charabanc driver.

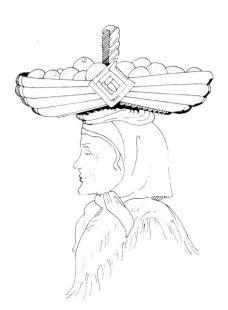

Head-pad worn for carrying in the 20th century.

Doormen, porters and page boys belonging to clubs and public buildings also frequently wore navy, though dark green and maroon were used as well for liveries modelled upon those of servants in private households. In most instances their coats, jackets and peaked caps were ornamented with braid, sometimes with epaulettes and buttons. For pages the buttons were round and set in two or three rows down the chest. (*Plate 28, fig. 137.*) Doormen often wore a top-hat with a cockade reminiscent of the previous century.

There were still footmen in private service and they and other English servants were much sought after and highly paid in wealthy American households. Livery, even there, was as elaborate as ever. Although trousers were considered quite appropriate for informal occasions, usually when there were less than twelve for dinner, breeches were used at other times. In less ostentatious houses, however, butler and footman dressed alike in black tail-coats and either striped or black trousers. Waiters also wore black coats and trousers, while chefs now dressed entirely in white and had acquired their tall 'cauliflower' hats. (*Plate 28, fig. 138.*)

Although coloured cotton or linen dresses were correct in the mornings for maidservants of all kinds to wear with their plain caps and aprons, in the afternoons parlourmaids and the new hybrids, house-parlourmaids, wore plain black dresses with fashionably short skirts and frilled or lace-edged white aprons. (*Plate 28, fig. 136.*)

Fishermen, though they might wear oilskins when at sea, usually favoured short smock-like garments of either brown or blue canvas or denim, or a combination of both colours. (*Plate 27, fig. 132.*) Under these they wore heavy woollen jerseys and coarse trousers. Many of the jerseys were home-knitted and had intricate patterns which were often associated with a specific area, or even with a particular family, frequently serving as a means of identifying men who had been drowned. Jerseys were worn, too, by sailors employed by shipping lines whose initials might be embroidered on the front. Sou'westers (oilskin hats with brims longer at the back than the front) were also a part of fishermen's dress.

Among the professional classes the wig had been retained for court use in a short and a long form by barristers and judges, in spite of the fact that it had been out of fashion for general wear since the end of the eighteenth century. In England this tradition has continued up to the present time.

As the story of occupational dress draws near to modern times, it can be seen that though some of the clothes, like the blacksmith's leather apron (*Plate 27, fig. 131*) had remained virtually unaltered for centuries, the post-war period was one in which workers dressed very similarly to their employers; only poverty, uniform, or garments added for a particular purpose, set them apart. In Sunday best there was little distinction, apart from taste. Two factors had helped to bring this about: improvement in earnings and the increased output of ready-to-wear clothes.

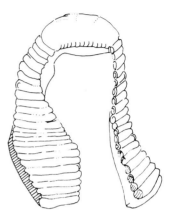

20th-century judge's wig.

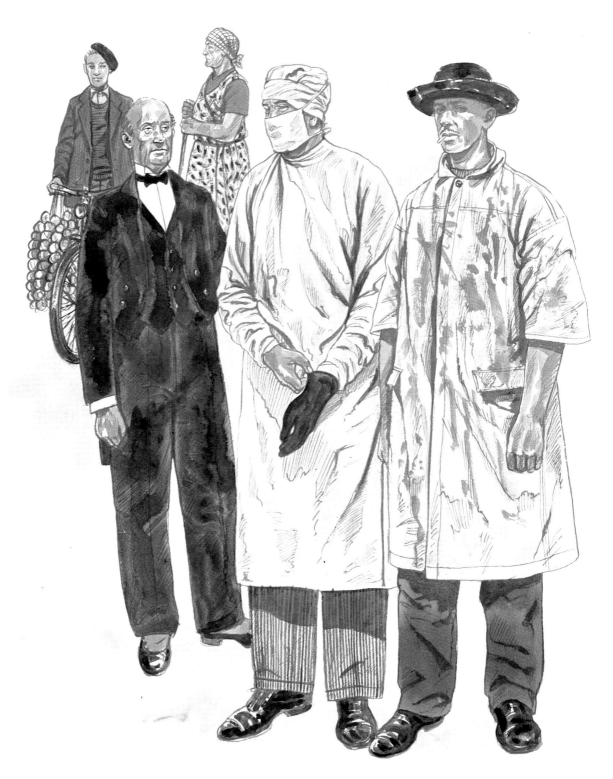

Plate 32   Chapter 10—late 1930's—England   (*Back left*) *Fig. 156* Onion boy (Itinerant trader from France), (*Front right*) *Fig. 157* Charwoman, (*Front left*) *Fig. 158* Butler, (*Centre front*) *Fig. 159* Surgeon in theatre dress, (*Front right*) *Fig. 160* Fish porter (Billingsgate Market, London).

10 White collar, blue collar, and no collar at all

1925–1939

ALTHOUGH THERE WAS A VAST AMOUNT of unemployment in Europe and North America in the 1920s and 1930s, the majority of workers were better dressed and followed fashion more closely than ever before. Newspaper, advertising and the cinema kept them up-to-date, while mass production made clothes readily available.

While in general everyone had some fashionable garments, there still remained differences between basic working dress and that of a few occupations. Most notable were those between the working clothes of what are often referred to as white-collar workers and blue-collar workers, differences that were to a large extent social rather than occupational. In the widest sense the distinction was, of course, in the collar itself, as the name suggests, but occupation and position were also indicated by the type of head-gear, by the removal or retention of the jacket and by the use of aprons.

Broadly speaking, basic working dress was the style of the period according to what the worker could afford. Those who did not use basic working dress were either provided with uniform or with protective clothing. (*Plate 32, fig. 160.*)

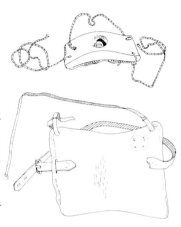

20th-century wood-worker's side apron (left) and breast pad (right).

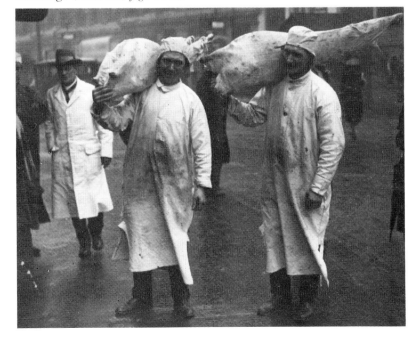

Porters at London's Smithfield Market wearing their new hygienic protective caps and 'smocks', or overalls. (1925)

The number of uniformed workers had greatly increased. A regulation style of dress had been found to be good publicity for the employer and a valuable prerequisite for the wearer, while increasing pressure was being brought to bear for the provision of protective clothing. In these two types of clothes lie the occupational, as distinct from the social, differences in working clothes for the years before the Second World War.

There was now less to choose between the fabrics worn by the various classes: corduroy was not so widely used by working men as it had been, tweed and woollen cloth having taken its place to a great extent. The jacket, of similar material to the trousers, was usually discarded by blue-collar workers and the waistcoat often replaced by a sleeveless woollen pullover, though some men wore shirt and trousers only. In England it was still very unusual for the shirt to be left off altogether, even in the hottest weather. Shirts, on which the place of the collar was taken by a knotted handkerchief or a muffler, were usually of striped cotton or flannel. White-collar workers, of course, retained collar, tie and waistcoat and, in some occupations, jacket as well. Boots tended to be worn by the labourer and shoes by others. Where uniform caps were not provided cloth caps were usual, but at the end of the period trilbys

Racing drivers and mechanics wearing different types and colours of boiler suits to protect their ordinary clothes. (1928)

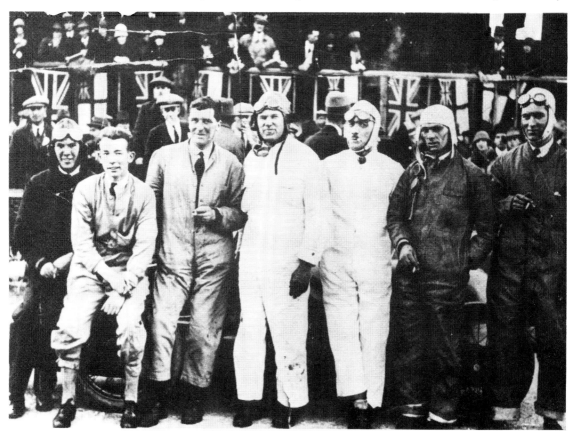

were often used by craftsmen in place of the bowler hats they had previously favoured.

Although not a type of protective clothing provided by the employer, bib-and-brace overalls were much worn by those working with machinery and, gradually, these became a symbol of manual labour. A mural at the New York World Fair of 1939 depicted a typical worker as wearing these 'dungarees', a short-sleeved shirt similar to the T-shirt of today, and gauntleted gloves.

Protective gloves were now used by a number of occupations and, as similar additions were common to several of them, it becomes difficult to be specific.

By the middle of the 1920s most of the older styles of occupational dress had vanished, including the countryman's smock, while some new ones had arrived, like the waterproof tabards worn by street cleaners, and the hard hats with lamps that were used by miners.

For most country workers rubber boots were now the usual footwear, replacing hob-nailed boots and the various kinds of leg protection previously used. Although shepherds, finding these boots too hot for a long day away from home, kept to gaiters that could be removed if the weather grew warm and dry. Advertisements of the time offer farm

Coal miners lightly clad to keep cool underground, but wearing protective helmets and leg pads. (1934)

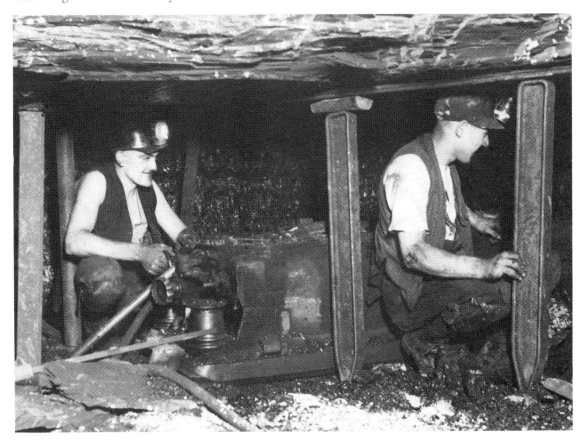

131

workers 'work oilskins' and sou'westers but most made do with old jackets, waistcoats and trousers which they tucked into their boots to obtain, once again, the convenience of breeches. A popular and effective covering was a sack, with either holes cut for head and arms or simply folded and put on like a hood to protect head and back. (*Plate 30, fig. 149.*) Gloves and knee pads were still used for special tasks like hedging, ditching, and thatching.

Farmers of the period, not wishing to look like their farm hands, often wore riding breeches and boots, or gaiters, with bowler hats rather than caps.

Country women doing farm work wore dresses, or blouses, with the addition of an apron or a sleeveless overall. The wrap-across patterned overall was typical working dress in the 'thirties. (*Plate 32, fig. 157.*) Sun-bonnets were used for harvesting and fruit picking. There were still a few groups of bondagers (*see* chapter 7) who clung to their traditional dress of coloured blouse, dark skirt and dark apron with the distinctive lined straw hat worn over a cotton head scarf. Like many other workers of the period, these women sometimes made use of army surplus garments, winding khaki puttees round their legs to take the place of gaiters. (*Plate 30, fig. 147.*)

The clothes of factory workers now varied according to the type of job they did. Ordinary male working dress of shirt, trousers, with pullover or waistcoat, and a cloth cap was common, though bib-and-brace overalls or boiler suits were worn when machinery was involved. In heavy industry a wide range of protective garments were added. Welders, for instance, in addition to their boiler suits, had knee pads, goggles and gloves.

Women in factories either wore the sleeveless overall or coat-overall, usually with a cap. (*Plate 30, fig. 150.*) Some factories supplied overalls of different colours for each department to make it easy to trace workers who moved away from their allotted places.

Many firms now had fleets of lorries and these were often driven by men in livery who, like porters and carriers for centuries, wore metal badges bearing their number. These liveries invariably included peaked caps and gaiters but might consist either of an overcoat with leather collar and cuffs (*Plate 29, fig. 143*), or the jacket and breeches of the private chauffeur.

Motor traffic of all kinds had greatly increased and many navvies had to be employed to keep the roads in order. Generally these men replaced the waistcoat with the knitted sleeveless pullover, otherwise their dress of cap, woollen shirt, heavy boots, and trousers tied below the knee, was unaltered. (*Plate 29, fig. 145.*)

In some cities street traders dressed in jacket and trousers with cloth caps and mufflers still sold goods from barrows. (*Plate 31, fig. 151.*) Another familiar sight in England during this period was the French

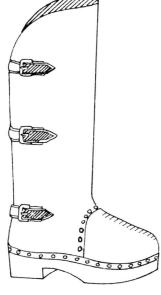

Butcher's washing clogs, 20th century.

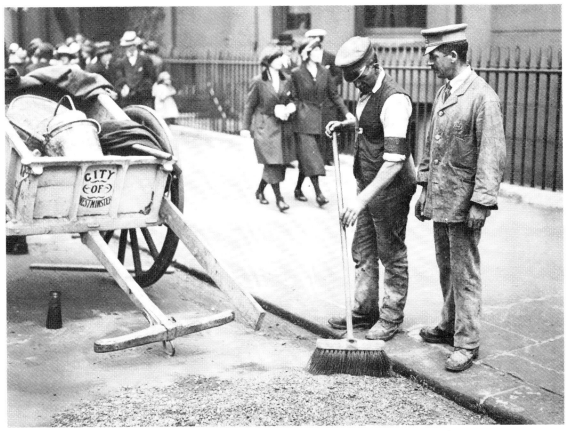

onion boy with his black beret and corduroy jacket. (*Plate 32, fig. 156.*)

Most milkmen now had trolleys which they pushed from behind and, even in 1938, they might still be seen in breeches and leather gaiters, with dark jackets and peaked caps, though some adopted trousers with white jackets or blue-and-white-striped aprons. Bread delivery men, who also sometimes had trolleys, wore ordinary working dress with waistcoats and white bibless aprons. (*Plate 31, fig. 152.*)

Fawn overalls had now largely relaced the shopman's long white apron though in the better food shops, particularly in cities, white coat-overalls and aprons were used. In small shops the white bibless apron was worn with suit collar and tie. (*Plate 29, fig. 141.*) Aprons were sometimes fastened to a waistcoat button in the middle of the chest. Most butchers continued to wear blue-and-white-striped aprons with white coat-overalls and, if a shop was open-fronted or goods displayed outside, the straw boater. Waterproof aprons were used by fishmongers as well as striped aprons. Waterproof materials were also appropriate for the messier butchery operations while heavy wooden-soled clogs with leggings attached were used by slaughterers.

Carpenters, considering themselves craftsmen, tended to be white-

City of Westminster foreman wearing a uniform jacket and trousers with a workman in corduroy waistcoat and trousers. Both men have dark blue peaked caps. (1925)

collar workers and wear shirt, waistcoat and tie, with a white, bibbed apron held round the neck with a loop. Joiners preferred light brown, or fawn, button-through coat-overalls. Bricklayers seldom bothered to put anything over ordinary working dress but, as they worked out of doors, wore hats, usually trilbys. Tradition still kept removal men in bowler hats and green baize aprons, while blacksmiths had found no more efficient protection from the heat of the forge than the ancient leather apron with a split up the centre.

Several new occupations for both men and women had grown out of the cinema industry. Films were shown in what were aptly named 'picture palaces' and, as was to be expected in palaces, visitors were treated with ceremony by attendants in elaborate livery. Commission-aires wore long coats in rich colours trimmed with metal buttons and braid, while the ushers inside wore colourful versions of footmen's livery jackets and trousers. (*Plate 31. figs. 153 and 154.*) Women ushers, or usherettes, had skirts and military-style jackets in similar rich colours, also with braid and buttons.

Far more people were using restaurants and there had been a con-siderable increase in moderately-priced eating places where waitresses were now more often employed than waiters. Most were provided by their employers with black long-sleeved dresses, small white aprons, caps and cuffs. (*Plate 29. fig. 142.*) This also remained the dress of the parlourmaid in private houses. Due to the difficulty of finding domes-tic servants, parlourmaids were now often called house-parlourmaids and expected to combine their own work with that of a housemaid. Cooks also had to do housework and were frequently referred to as cook-generals. The shortage of domestic staff was partly due to the conditions under which many still worked but also to an increasing distaste for the servility of cap and apron. Some employers attempted to alleviate this by providing dresses of blue, green or brown instead of the dreary black, and aprons and caps in beige or contrasting pastel shades. Others improved the quality of the clothes themselves, even to the extent of giving their maids tussore silk to wear in summer. Nevertheless, the discontent with cap and apron grew and plain white or coloured overalls began to be used instead.

Although more people now drove their own cars, chauffeurs were employed in the larger establishments and still dressed, as previously, in livery jackets, breeches and gaiters. Gradually, however, many adopted easy-fitting jackets and trousers, though the peaked cap (worn with a white cover in summer) and leather gloves continued. Heavy coats were not so essential as most cars were saloons.

In general a more democratic attitude towards domestic service now existed and there was less ostentation; elaborately dressed servants were no longer used as a means of displaying wealth. Footmen still remained but rarely wore breeches, dressing similarly to the butler in his black tail-coat, black trousers, hard shirt and grey spats. (*Plate 32. fig. 158.*) For informal wear pantry jackets, or sleeved waistcoats with striped fronts, replaced the tail-coat.

Although grooms seldom wore livery, jerseys and riding breeches with tweed jackets being usual, the silk shirts and breeches of jockeys and their peaked caps recalled the grooms' dress of the past, as well as being a lingering example of an employee carrying his master's colours on his back. (*Plate 30. fig. 146.*)

Many workers now wore uniforms of dark jackets and trousers, styles varying according to the organization and to the status of the worker. The differences were usually apparent in the jacket and in the head-gear; railway porters and ticket collectors had sleeved waistcoats and short jackets respectively with different types of peaked caps, while station masters of main line stations wore top-hats, usually with morning dress or long black overcoats.

The peaked cap had space in front for a badge and carried with it an official air that the cloth cap did not possess. It was frequently used as an official insignia by firms who supplied their employees with no other distinguishing uniform.

English postmen, in dark blue like many other countries, still had a trace of the old royal red livery in the piping on their trousers while their double peaked caps had been entirely replaced by caps with a single front peak. Bus and tram companies also had uniforms carefully graded according to rank but the drivers of the huge motors called charabancs, a popular form of transport for group outings, usually wore ordinary suits with peaked caps. (*Plate 31. fig. 155.*)

The dress of fishermen had not altered, though oilskins had some-what improved. Black ones were usually worn by pilots. (*Plate 30. fig. 148.*) Lifeboatmen replaced cork life jackets with ones made of canvas and kapok, using yellow as it was more easily seen. The diving suit of the deep-sea diver had not changed very much, apart from the impor-tant development that now enabled them to carry their air supply themselves instead of being dependent upon it being pumped from the surface.

By the end of the 1930s, lounge suits, either pin-striped or of plain material, were taking the place of morning dress for business; although bowler hats were still worn, the trilby and other forms of the felt hat were now acceptable.

Depending upon their jobs, women office workers used either tailor-made suits, plain dresses or blue overalls. (*Plate 29. fig. 144.*) Protec-tive oversleeves were also worn by both men and women clerks.

White jackets or coat overalls were now common for dentists and doctors in hospitals and clinics, while surgeons in the operating theatre had white overalls that fastened at the back to prevent the ties getting in the way. With the overalls they wore caps, masks and sterile rubber

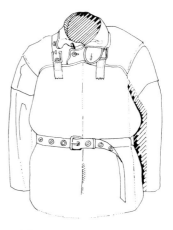

20th-century
lifeboatman's life-jacket.

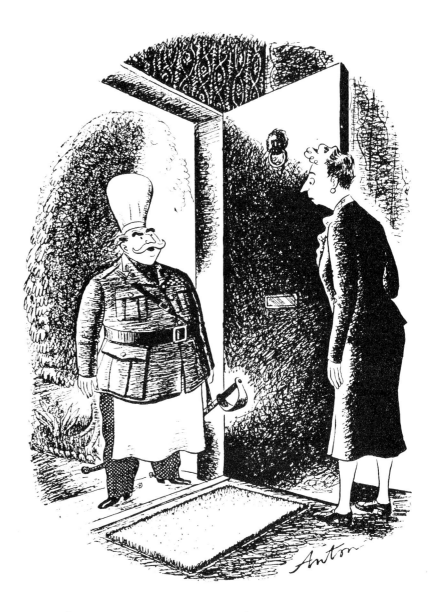

"ARE YOU THE LADY WHO'S ADVERTISING FOR A COOK-GENERAL?"

gloves which were intended not to protect them so much as to avoid any infection being passed to the patient. (*Plate 32, fig. 159.*)

Throughout all professions white shirts with black jackets and trousers, or morning dress with striped trousers, were still considered appropriate, and hats and gloves were always worn in the street. In court judges and barristers used gowns and wigs for the same reasons that long robes had been worn by the learned in Medieval times, to give dignity and authority.

This clinging to the fashions of earlier times can be seen in other working clothes of the 'thirties, though for different reasons. The blacksmith's leather aprons, for instance, had hardly altered since it was used in ancient Greece and Rome; white bibless aprons had been working wear since the Middle Ages; and the tying of trousers below the knee by labourers was an attempt to return to the convenience of eighteenth-century breeches. The continental workman's loose blouse followed the pattern of the ancient tunic with sleeves; while the older sleeveless version is reflected in the use of sacks with holes cut for head and arms. Sacks recall the Medieval hood when folded in half and worn over the head.

Right up to modern times occupational accessories recall the past. Today, boards are still attached to the feet to prevent them sinking in mud or sand; eye-shields, goggles and bee-veils, though they may be made of different materials, closely resemble those used centuries ago. Nowhere has necessity been more the mother of invention than in occupational costume.

Attitudes may have changed and standardization taken over but the requirements of the worker have not altered: it is still necessary to have clothes that are suitable for the job while preserving decency and offering protection.

Thus, although the picturesque aspects of occupational costume, which must have brightened many otherwise dreary lives, may have gone for ever, the basics are, and will continue, the same. In occupational costume, as in many other things, the more it changes the more it remains the same.

Further Reading

Arnold, J. *A Handbook of Costume* Macmillan, 1973

Boucher, F. *A History of Costume in the West* Thames and Hudson, 1967

Buck, A. *Dress in Eighteenth Century England* Batsford, 1979

Byrde, P. *The Male Image* Batsford, 1979

Copeland, P. F. *Working Dress in Colonial and Revolutionary America* Greenwood Press, 1977

Cunnington, P. and Lucas, C. *Occupational Costume in England, from the 11th Century to 1914* A. & C. Black, 1967

Davenport, M. *The Book of Costume* Crown Publishers, New York, 1948

Landsell, A. *Occupational Costume* Shire Album No. 27, 1977

Oakes, A. and Hill, M. H. *Rural Costume, its Origin and Development in Western Europe and the British Isles* Batsford, 1970

Illustration Credits

The colour plates are painted by Jeffrey J. Burn and the line drawings are by Christine Taylor. The publishers would like to thank the following for their permission to reproduce the black and white pictures on the pages mentioned:

By gracious permission of H.M. the Queen   32, 67, 74
British Library   20, 22, 24, 34, 49
Cambridge University Library   35
Chertsey Museum   122
Christies   47
Exeter Museums   71
Faith Legg   103, 106
Mansell Collection   50, 51
Mary Evans Picture Library   57, 84
Christobel Williams-Mitchell   109
Museum of English Rural Life   55
Phaidon Press   17
Popper Photos   104, 105
Punch   136
Radio Times Hulton Picture Library   14, 42, 43, 88, 89, 92, 97
114, 115, 123, 129, 131, 133
Royal National Lifeboat Institution   99
Victoria and Albert Museum   32
Weybridge Museum   119, 130
Gordon Winter   100, 102

Index

Numbers in **bold type** refer to colour plates; **5**(23), for example, indicates Plate 5, Figure 23. Page numbers in *italics* refer to the black-and-white illustrations.